DREAMS OF A HEALTHY INDIA

Celebrating 35 Years of
Penguin Random House India

RETHINKING INDIA
Series editors: Aakash Singh Rathore, Mridula Mukherjee,
Pushparaj Deshpande and Syeda Hameed

OTHER BOOKS IN THE SERIES
Vision for a Nation: Paths and Perspectives
(Aakash Singh Rathore and Ashis Nandy, eds)

The Minority Conundrum: Living in Majoritarian Times
(Tanweer Fazal, ed.)

Reviving Jobs: An Agenda for Growth
(Santosh Mehrotra, ed.)

We the People: Establishing Rights and Deepening Democracy
(Nikhil Dey, Aruna Roy and Rakshita Swamy, eds)

The Shudras: Vision for a New Path
(Kancha Ilaiah Shepherd and Karthik Raja Karuppusamy, eds)

Her Right to Equality: From Promise to Power
(Nisha Agrawal, ed.)

Being Adivasi: Existence, Entitlements, Exclusion
(Abhay Flavian Xaxa and G.N. Devy, eds)

The Dalit Truth: The Battles for Realizing Ambedkar's Vision
(K. Raju, ed.)

RETHINKING INDIA

DREAMS OF A HEALTHY INDIA

DEMOCRATIC HEALTH CARE IN POST-COVID TIMES

Edited by

RITU PRIYA
SYEDA HAMEED

VINTAGE
An imprint of Penguin Random House

VINTAGE

USA | Canada | UK | Ireland | Australia
New Zealand | India | South Africa | China

Vintage is part of the Penguin Random House group of companies
whose addresses can be found at global.penguinrandomhouse.com

Published by Penguin Random House India Pvt. Ltd
4th Floor, Capital Tower 1, MG Road,
Gurugram 122 002, Haryana, India

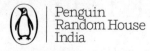

Penguin
Random House
India

First published in Vintage by Penguin Random House India 2023

ISBN 9780670093021

Typeset in Bembo Std by Manipal Technologies Limited, Manipal
Printed at Thomson Press India Ltd, New Delhi

www.penguin.co.in

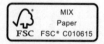

*Dedicated to the front-line workers who served during the
COVID-19 pandemic, even at risk to their lives*

*To those who strive in 'normal' times to promote
health and prevent ill-health*

*To those who devote themselves to health of their families
and communities in harmony with nature*

To those who serve 'insaniyat' with love

'Maqam-e-shauq tere qudisyon ke bas mein nahin
Unhi ka kaam hai ye jinke hausley hain buland'

*(The station of love is beyond the reach of your angels
Only those with dauntless courage can achieve it)*

—Allama Iqbal

Contents

Series Editors' Note

Psychologists tell us that the only true enemies we have are the faces looking back at us in the mirror. Today, we in India need to take a long, hard look at ourselves in the mirror. With either actual or looming crises in every branch of government, at every level, be it central, state or local; with nearly every institution failing; with unemployment at historically high rates; with an ecosystem ready to implode; with a health-care system in a shambles; with an education system on the brink of collapse; with gender, caste and class inequities unabating; with civil society increasingly characterized by exclusion, intolerance and violence; with our own minorities living in fear; our hundreds of millions of fellow citizens in penury; and with few prospects for the innumerable youth of this nation in the face of all these increasingly intractable problems, the reflection is not sightly. Our true enemies are not external to us, not Pakistani terrorists or Bangladeshi migrants, but our own selves: our own lack of imagination, communication, cooperation and dedication towards achieving the India of our destiny and dreams.

Our Constitution, as the Preamble so eloquently attests, was founded upon the fundamental values of the dignity of the individual and the unity of the nation, envisioned in relation to a radically egalitarian justice. These bedrock ideas, though perhaps especially pioneered by the likes of Jawaharlal Nehru, B.R. Ambedkar, M.K. Gandhi, Maulana Azad, Sardar Patel, Sarojini Naidu, Jagjivan Ram, R. Amrit Kaur, Ram Manohar Lohia and others, had emerged as a broad consensus among the many founders of this nation, cutting across divergent social and political ideologies. Giving shape to that vision, the architects of modern India strived to ensure that each one of us is accorded equal opportunities to live with dignity and security, has equitable access to a better life, and is an equal partner in this nation's growth.

Yet, today we find these most basic constitutional principles under attack. Nearly all the public institutions that were originally created in order to fight against dominance and subservience are in the process of subversion, creating new hierarchies instead of dismantling them, generating inequities instead of ameliorating them. Government policy merely pays lip service to egalitarian considerations, while the actual administration of 'justice' and implementation of laws are in fact perpetuating precisely the opposite: illegality, criminality, corruption, bias, nepotism and injustice of every conceivable stripe. And the rapid rise of social intolerance and manifold exclusions (along the lines of gender, caste, religion, etc.) effectively whittle down and even sabotage an inclusive conception of citizenship, polity and nation.

In spite of these and all the other unmentioned but equally serious challenges posed at this moment, there are in fact new sites for socio-political assertion re-emerging. There are new calls arising for the reinstatement of the letter and spirit of our Constitution, not just normatively (where we battle things out ideologically) but also practically (the battle at the level of policy articulation and implementation). These calls are not simply partisan, nor are they exclusionary or zero-sum. They witness the wide participation of youth, women, the historically disadvantaged in the process of finding a new voice, minorities, members of majority communities, and progressive individuals all joining hands in solidarity.

We at the Samruddha Bharat Foundation proudly count ourselves among them. The Foundation's very raison d'être has been to take serious cognizance of India's present and future challenges, and to rise to them. Over the past two years, we have constituted numerous working groups to critically rethink social, economic and political paradigms to encourage a transformative spirit in India's polity. Over 400 of India's foremost academics, activists, professionals and policymakers across party lines have constructively engaged in this process. We have organized and assembled inputs from *jan sunwais* (public hearings) and *jan manchs* (public platforms) that we conducted across several states, and discussed and debated these ideas with leaders of fourteen progressive political parties, in an effort to set benchmarks for a future common minimum programme. The overarching idea has been to try to breathe new life and spirit into the cold and self-serving logic of political and administrative processes, linking them to and informing them by grassroots realities, fact-based research and social experience, and actionable social–scientific knowledge. And to do all of this with harmony and heart, with sincere emotion and national feeling.

In order to further disseminate these ideas, both to kick-start a national dialogue and to further build a consensus on them, we are bringing out this set of fourteen volumes highlighting innovative ideas that seek to deepen and further the promise of India. This is not an academic exercise; we do not merely spotlight structural problems, but also propose disruptive solutions to each of the pressing challenges that we collectively face. All the essays, though authored by top academics, technocrats, activists, intellectuals and so on, have been written purposively to be accessible to a general audience, whose creative imagination we aim to spark and whose critical feedback we intend to harness, leveraging it to further our common goals.

The inaugural volume has been specifically dedicated to our norms, to serve as a fresh reminder of our shared and shareable overlapping values and principles, collective heritage and resources.

Titled *Vision for a Nation: Paths and Perspectives*, it champions a plural, inclusive, just, equitable and prosperous India, and is committed to individual dignity, which is the foundation of the unity and vibrancy of the nation.

The thirteen volumes that follow turn from the normative to the concrete. From addressing the problems faced by diverse communities—adivasis, Dalit Bahujans, other backward classes (OBCs)—as well as women and minorities, to articulating the challenges that we face with respect to jobs and unemployment, urbanization, health care and a rigged economy, to scrutinizing our higher education system or institutions more broadly, each volume details some ten specific policy solutions promising to systemically treat the issue(s), transforming the problem at a lasting structural level, not just a superficial one. These innovative and disruptive policy solutions flow from the authors' research, knowledge and experience, but they are especially characterized by their unflinching commitment to our collective normative understanding of who we can and ought to be.

The volumes that look at the concerns, needs and aspirations of the Shudras, Dalits, adivasis and women particularly look at how casteism has played havoc with India's development and stalled the possibility of the progressive transformation of Indian society. They first analyse how these sections of society have faced historical and structural discrimination against full participation in Indian spiritual, educational, social and political institutions for centuries. They also explore how the reforms that some of our epoch-making socio-political thinkers like Gautama Buddha, M.K. Gandhi, Jawaharlal Nehru and B.R. Ambedkar foregrounded are being systematically reversed by regressive forces and the ruling elite because of their ideological proclivities. These volumes therefore strive to address some of the most glaring social questions that India faces from a modernist perspective and propose a progressive blueprint that will secure spiritual, civil and political liberties for one and all.

What the individual volumes aim to offer, then, are navigable road maps for how we may begin to overcome the many specific challenges that we face, guiding us towards new ways of working cooperatively to rise above our differences, heal the wounds in our communities, recalibrate our modes of governance and revitalize our institutions. Cumulatively, however, they achieve something of even greater synergy, greater import: they reconstruct that India of our imagination, of our aspirations, the India reflected in the constitutional preamble that we all surely want to be a part of.

Let us put aside that depiction of a mirror with an enemy staring back at us. Instead, together, we help to construct a whole new set of images. One where you may look at your nation and see your individual identity and dignity reflected in it, and when you look within your individual self, you may find the pride of your nation residing there.

Aakash Singh Rathore, Mridula Mukherjee,
Pushparaj Deshpande and *Syeda Hameed*

Preface

This volume on 'Dreams of a Healthy India', part of the Rethinking India series, comes at a time when the COVID pandemic has foregrounded health, health care and health systems as issues of critical importance in the public mind. It has brought home the significance of the public system as the major source of health-care activities for disease control and medical care. At a time when the private sector was being considered the more efficient provider of quality health care, this has led to interest in the upgrading of public-health systems. At the same time, the pandemic has also given added salience to people's own self-care and access to medical care from home. The COVID-generated crisis has, thus, led to an enhanced interest in the contents of this volume.

This volume is an attempt to demystify the issues of health care and health systems for the general reader, as well as to simultaneously provoke rethinking on several critical dimensions by policymakers and academics. Its introductory essay and the thirteen subsequent essays lay out the scenario as well as the challenges and then provide doable solutions. These are solutions for the present times that can simultaneously contribute to sustainable health care for the future. Cast in an accessible style, these essays present the challenges of the current scenario in all its varied hues. Complex ideas are not made simplistic but are presented in simple language, with some illustrative case studies and vignettes or data that speaks for itself.

As editors of the volume, we believe that there has to be a rethink on the popular image of health care as merely medical care alone. Also, a rethink about the nineteenth- and twentieth-century image of hospitals and health centres that we still seem to work with. Systemic issues, such as of increasing doctor–patient distrust, of plural health knowledge systems, need to be understood with scientific rigour and dealt with in the collaborative spirit of the twenty-first century. Forums for dialogue will have to be institutionalized across the diverse actors and interests within the health system. But for that to be meaningfully possible, issues of health care and health systems have to be understood and engaged with by a much wider section of the concerned public. Their contribution to the designing of creative and contextually appropriate models of health care is the way forward. That scientific temper can go together with plural medicine and create more effective health care, that small community hospitals can provide tertiary levels of medical care, that decentralized health research can be carried out to find local best solutions for health problems, all these are ideas that need a societal rethink.

To policymakers and academics, this volume presents ideas that respond to the needs of all in a sustainable way; that are essential for the making of an inclusive and democratic Indian vision of health care for the twenty-first century. Several policy issues of health care and institutional design of health systems have remained areas of dissonance and tension over the decades. Most of the essays here address one or more of such areas and present ways of resolving the issues with better coherence. The ideas for futuristic development presented in each essay have evolved from grounded experience and successful application in concrete form. The essays present them as critical correctives that require a rethink and change of mindset. Despite the diverse disciplinary, theoretical and ideological moorings of the authors, together the ideas across these essays add up to a new vision of what a contextually appropriate, sustainable health system can look like and how to make it happen.

Introduction

Transforming Indian Health Care: Towards Sustainable and Empowering Systems

Ritu Priya and Syeda Hameed

Y ou are an exceptionally lucky Indian if you have a trustworthy doctor to turn to. You are equally lucky if you have gained full height, do not suffer from daily aches and pains, are not wracked by bouts of acute respiratory illnesses or other more chronic conditions. These common ailments afflict a vast majority of Indians, and frequently spiral into crippling crises for individuals and families.

It's ironic that a nation that aspires to be a global superpower pays so little heed to empowering its citizens for ensuring their wellbeing, to guarantee what India's first prime minister so poetically characterized as fullness of life. This is when India has grown from being a 'low-income country' to a 'middle-income country', with economic growth rates outpacing those of most nations. Our doctors and nurses have become a mainstay of the American, British and other nations' health services. Yet in India, there is a massive 'trust deficit' between doctors, hospitals, the overall health system and the public. Our states consistently rank low on global health and health-care indicators[1]. And most problematically of all, a shocking 2.4 million (24 lakh) Indians die of treatable conditions *every year*.[2] Why are we so sanguine about the wellbeing of our fellow Indians, and indeed face the consequences as we did during the COVID-19 waves? And why are we so tolerant towards this abysmal state of affairs?

Bordering on a national cliche, it is widely felt that government health-care services in India are inadequate in terms of number of centres and hospitals, as well as the number of doctors and other personnel in them. We also know that private-sector health services are profit-making entities, and are widely perceived to engage in malpractices of over-prescription and over-charging.[3] Exacerbating matters, there is a massive information asymmetry between service providers and the users, which adds to a trust deficit. Yet, we do nothing until a health crisis affects someone close to us.

On the flip side, it is equally true that the health services system, with both public and private constituents, is not satisfactory from the perspective of most health-care providers either, since work conditions do not provide for professional satisfaction in patient care. After all, it is the system in which doctors get placed that shapes their behaviour and the services they provide. The public system is hamstrung by inadequate facilities while the private system faces immense pressure from hospital management and commercial interests for over-medicalization. This over-medicalization is sometimes also the result of patient/relative demand, since they have become habituated to unnecessary, irrational overuse of diagnostics, medicines and medical interventions. Administrators in the public system are constrained by the resources at hand, while private hospital managements are under pressure to put in place capital-intensive infrastructure and install the latest technologies, while being burdened by high running costs and the owner/shareholders' demand for profits.

If we are to transform health care in India, we need to first recognize the systemic nature of the health-care crisis. Every stakeholder—the users, providers and managers are struggling to bandage structural fault lines. Clearly, a major surgery is needed.

But individual health is not shaped solely by the medical care we can access or an individual's genetic attributes. It is shaped by the systems that mould us—our environment, food, living and work patterns, social relationships, emotional state and our health-care-related practices.[4] Every day, we make choices related to these variables that impact our health, whether it is our diet, our clothes, our sleep, our leisure activities and so on.

Despite the inter-connectedness of individual and systemic variables in shaping our health care, 'health' has not gained the public salience to merit collective thinking or mobilization on an appreciable scale. Health care is still relegated as an area for individuals to muddle though as best as they can when they are ill. Additionally, it is considered too technical, and therefore not engaged with by most Indians as a serious policy issue.

When down with an illness, we choose from the health services available, and manage with whatever is best suited for us. In such a time of crisis, firefighting is the priority—not deciding on ways to improve and strengthen the various choices in health care or generate public pressure for the same. Later, we get busy with other things. Or we scapegoat individual doctors, rather than underscore the limitations that ail the system. This ignoring of systemic and collective causes of ill-health is certainly at our own peril, as individuals and as a society.

Dilemmas and Dreams for a Healthy India: Systemic Innovations

India is set to be the biggest and youngest nation on the planet in the remaining three-quarters of the twenty-first century. With the largest number of young people, India could provide the workforce for the global economy, and reap demographic dividends. However, the opposite is also likely—that India will have an ageing population that struggles with chronic illnesses while the children and workforce age-group struggle with lack of access to early diagnosis and care for acute health conditions, ending up with an earlier onset of chronic illnesses. Ensuring that India is on track to being healthy, happy and productive will require a serious consideration of the current situation and putting in place a series of measures to enable the realization of this dream.

Health policy concerns, articulated in pre-COVID times, will now additionally have to contend with the need for preparedness to deal with future pandemics. The COVID-19 pandemic demonstrated that we have primary-level public health services in all states and union territories that can be mobilized at the ground level—visible in efforts at contract tracing and testing and following up on people testing positive, and the extent of vaccination that was accomplished once adequate vaccine stocks became available. But it was only in some states that this primary-level care could be considered reasonably satisfactory in coverage and quality. It was again public hospitals that provided a major part of the hospital care required for moderately or seriously ill COVID-19 cases. Doctors, nurses, paramedical and support staff all performed a humungous task over the two years we experienced of the pandemic, going well beyond their call of duty. Yet, even in normal times, our public hospitals are not the most patient-friendly of places.

Is it that we are so resource-constrained that we cannot develop an adequate health-care system for all Indians? Is it that the inequalities in access to incomes, material goods and services are so wide that most Indians remain deprived, while only the better off get good quality, trustworthy health care? Or is it also that the kind of system we have attempted to develop for ourselves has been unsuited to our context and to the provision of a societally affordable, inclusive, caring and humane service system?

Is a doctor- and hospital-centred imagination of health care the only one we can aspire to? Or should we view them as essential but partial components of what 'health care' is about? Can medical services be effective in improving a population's health if basic conditions of life are unhealthy?

COVID-19 has reminded us that human health is closely intertwined with ecology and economics. Whether the virus came from a laboratory or the wet market in Wuhan remains a matter of controversy. But in either case, it points to the breaking down of ecological barriers between viruses, which nature cloistered in remote niches, and the human species. The pandemic was the result of an interplay of factors: human initiatives focused on global chains for esoteric food, megalomanic notions of investigating such natural virus niches to generate technological solutions to pandemic control before the infection reaches us,[5] and the natural dynamics set up by the decreasing bio-diversity.[6] Clearly, human-centric and technology-centred approaches alone cannot protect human health. A healthy human environment requires a healthy ecological system, which includes the physical, biological and social. Can we envisage what can be called 'health-care habitats'—our living and working spaces as places that enhance rather than detract from our health and happiness? *The post-COVID world will have to decide what is to be the central focus of future development—economics or health. Health requires a balance of economic, technological and social development that caters to the wellbeing of humans and the planet.*

The variable quality and increasing iatrogenesis (ill-health effects of medical care) as well as the growing mutual distrust between health-care providers and the people must be actively addressed. What correctives are needed in our vision as well as in concrete action plans? How do we go beyond the present vision of health care as merely medical intervention? How do we knit together all the advances in the understanding of human health and its links with societal and environmental determinants, knowledge systems, technologies and policies, as well as people's action to build the healthy India of our dreams, with health care *for the people, of the people and by the people*?

Since health affects each one of us in the most personal and collective ways, as citizens, we need to be concerned about how our health-care system is shaped. To answer these questions, we need to think about what attributes we want to see in the health system. And, most importantly, how we can move towards mending what we have and adding value so that it meets our expectations.

Patterns of livelihood, distribution of material resources, social structures and value frames that are conducive to a culture of 'caring' will help us move towards our dream of a healthy India. Fostering a society of 'care' for human beings and nature is an essential element in resolving the civilizational crises today. That is what will lead to 'health-care habitats' and trustworthy health services. Caring for those with illness and suffering has always symbolized the most compassionate of human feelings and action, and health care is therefore central to the building of a caring society and State. Can we harness this two-way relationship between society and health-care systems to move towards the healthy India of our dreams?

We hope that this volume will contribute to demystifying the issues faced by health-care systems and initiate public discussion and action for inclusive, sustainable and people-empowering systems. The necessity of fulfilment of basic needs for a healthy population and the essential tenets of health-service systems, such as equity, accessibility, affordability, effectiveness, safety and quality, are widely known, but it is the feasibility of these desirables that is put to question in an imperfect world. It is the trade-offs that we choose, the systems we create for ourselves, that will decide our health and wellbeing, now and in the future. What systemic innovations can we devise that take health care in the country towards a societal value frame and capacitate it to meet the challenges of the twenty-first century?

In this volume, we attempt to make the systemic issues in health care accessible to the general reader. Each essay is by experts in the field of public health and health systems with a lifetime of work. The articles in Section I lay out the landscape that shapes health and health care and indicate directions to meet the challenges faced and build pathways towards creating a healthy people. They highlight for us the wider dimensions of health care, beyond the 'health sector' and the doctor- and hospital-centred image of what health care constitutes. In Section II, we present the contours of innovations to strengthen our health services for the twenty-first century. The essays here deal with some major dimensions of health services development and health governance. Since there are so many small and big innovations available in the practice of health care in India and globally, these essays can only illustrate some of them to indicate a coherent direction.

Demystifying Health Systems Development

Health systems research and policy studies is a vast and rapidly growing field of academic work and development practice. The present discipline can be considered to have started in the mid-nineteenth century, with the organizing of public service systems run by governments. The need for organized health care gained increasing significance in the twentieth century globally, with the world wars and newly independent countries shaking off colonial rule. Two broad strands of health systems development were evident, one that followed a top-down planning for delivering medical and health care, with some outreach community work, largely found in high-income countries and based on the Euro-American doctor-hospital model of the nineteenth and twentieth centuries. The other attempted to work upwards from the people's life conditions and context-specific health-care needs. As biomedicine grew and the medical industrial complex attempted to promote markets for its goods and services, the imagination of 'health care' became increasingly reduced to 'medical care'. This has led to only the top-down kind of health systems development becoming dominant in public imagination. The image of the best health care is that of big hospitals with the latest and most sophisticated medical technology. Do they provide the solution, or are they also part of the problem? The answer is not so white and black; hospitals play an important role in tertiary care, but a larger part of health care lies beyond them and needs a different imagination and approach for implementation.

Converting the principles of a bottoms-up approach, which goes back to people's life conditions, into real-life policies and plans and operationalizing the approaches considered appropriate is a complex political, administrative and human exercise. Systemic innovation lies in generating solutions to real-life problems affecting large sections of the population, by bringing together science, technology, human resources and delivery mechanisms in a way that they are best suited to the specific context to which they are to be applied. If learning from people's contexts—their health experiences, specific health-care-related perceptions, behaviours and practices—was part of the policymaking and systems design processes, would it not lead to more effective health systems development and better population health? There has been substantial application of the pro-people approach in India to thinking about health systems development, much research and experiments with it, many civil society initiatives providing a thrust. It is the grounded learnings from the experience of applying holistic approaches to health systems that this volume presents with hope and dreams for the future.

However, the dominant approach of health systems development has been doctor-and-hospital-centred. It has been counter-balanced to some extent by the pro-people approaches that raised dissenting voices and demonstrated other models than the dominant one. The debates in health systems development come from several unresolved issues. These include: defining 'health' and 'health care' to reflect their complexity in operational ways; identifying the role of medical and non-medical inputs in health care and thereby defining the contours of the 'health system' and what all health policy must attend to. Also, defining the place of conventional bio-medical 'modern' and 'traditional' health knowledges in the health system, and of expert (whether modern or traditional) and non-expert 'layperson' knowledge. Equally essential in considerations of health policy and systems design are the role of the public and private sectors in health care across the primary, secondary and tertiary levels of health care; the role of self-care and so on.

One of the related issues in health systems development has been the structure and processes of health governance; the systems of decision making and leadership. Centralized bureaucratic administrative structures at country level with internationalist knowledge centralization has been the dominant process. This is despite the constitutional mandate of health care being a state subject and structures for district- and local-level decentralized implementation and accountability. The decentralized approaches create diverse possibilities of responsiveness to the local context on the one hand and application of plural knowledge on the other. Therefore, administrative versus technical leadership and centralized versus decentralized decision-making structures have been contentious issues. In recent years this has further extended to creation of structures for regulating public-private partnerships, for instance in social insurance programmes such as Ayushman Bharat and the use of Digital Health data. The potential benefits of digital health data for each citizen requires health service systems that can access it when required. While this is a small advantage, it is meaningful for only a small segment of the population and with formal health services. Its danger is of authoritarian surveillance of individual behaviours in the name of health protection, with vigilance over individual lifestyle choices and coercion in consumption patterns, of food and commercial supplements for instance. Thereby, a careful balancing of the benefits and threats to peoples' health and wellbeing, transparency in administrative decision making and accountability to people is necessary, with consideration of new information technological tools and penetration of health care, pharmaceutical and corporate hospital industries. Intended and unintended consequences of the health-care systems we create now will affect several generations to come.

This volume addresses these debates and dilemmas of health care to argue that the approach that allows the most comprehensive, inclusive, democratic and pluralist system will be the most effective and sustainable. Technically stated, this would be an epidemiologically sound system, prioritizing attention to the pressing health problems of the most vulnerable sections and marginalized majorities, while holistically bridging the bottom-up and top-down perspectives with a 'complex adaptive systems' lens to design health policy and health-care systems for all.

As editors of this volume, we draw on our experience with health systems. A member of the Planning Commission with the portfolio of 'Health' over two terms (2004–2014), with a keen interest in women's health and minority issues, and engagement with civil society as an academic and writer, Syeda Hameed has come to understand health system debates of the time and also to appreciate the alternative system designs being implemented by civil society organizations that she has had occasion to visit. Ritu Priya, a medical graduate, a public health researcher and faculty at JNU since 1990, with a direct foray into government systems through a two-year stint at the National Health Systems Resource Centre (NHSRC) as adviser on Public Health Planning during the early years of implementation of the National Rural Health Mission (NRHM), has worked on health system issues in an academic capacity and as part of her engagement with central and state government agencies as well as with civil society groups. Our diverse trajectories have taught us the value of people-centred health care, of engaging with communities and planning for health well beyond the confines of the medical services alone.

So what follows in this introductory essay is our learnings from multiple sources and experiences—theoretical academic literature, insights and experiments on the ground, people we have interacted with, as well as the planning and institutional processes in the country. Based on our shared public- and community-centred approach to health care, we have invited authors to contribute essays on the various dimensions we considered relevant to spell out the dream of a healthy India and on innovative pathways to realize the dream.

In this introduction, we attempt to lay the ground for considering some of the unresolved questions, and briefly discuss the other essays in the volume that have been brought together to address the questions.

A Holistic Framework for Thinking about Health Care

What is 'Health'?

Health is about an active and 'normally' functioning body and mind, not merely absence of disease. It entails the capacity to withstand the physical and biological pressures of weather and climate, of infections entering the body, of toxins in the environment, of emotional disturbances and psychological tensions, of degenerative changes on account of ageing. These factors push one towards ill-health, and healthy people are those who are able to overcome such pressures and can bounce back to 'normal' functioning in accord with their age.

Health is a summary outcome of all the various dimensions that impinge on human wellbeing. This requires conditions of life that are supportive and facilitatory from womb to tomb. That is what is meant by population-level 'health care'. It not only includes arrangements for caring of the sick and treating disease as and when it occurs, but also much more in terms of the conditions of life. So, what is health care composed of?

What is Health Care?

What shapes people's health, individual and collective, is schematically depicted in the 'onion-peel' figure below. Beginning with People's Health as the core, by asking the 'what' question for each layer—'What shapes this?'—we get a systematic understanding of the 'causes of causes', and thereby the complexity of health and health care. It indicates to us what considerations are essential for people's physical and mental wellbeing, reiterating that health services are only one element in how society contributes to 'health care'.

The determinants of people's physical and mental health include the fulfilling of basic physical needs (*roti, kapda, makaan,* and in today's times, *bijli, pani, sadak, shiksha, rozgar, swasthya seva*), along with a sense of social and emotional wellbeing (that depends on the nature of social relationships) and spiritual wellbeing (that involves the sense of fulfilment and meaning in life). Since in the present world of nation states, governments are powerful in shaping people's material entitlements and their provisioning for all sections of society, public policy is of critical significance across sectors in shaping these conditions for population health. Public policies express societal priorities on one hand, and shape social value frames on the other. Affecting access to decent work and livelihoods, ecological integrity, social cohesion, and access to quality services, public policies lead to much more than just the specific material objectives for which they were intended. They contribute to a sense of identity, dignity and self-esteem in society, and influence the way people make life choices, including health-seeking behaviours. However, policies evolve through priority-setting; designing interventions and their implementation are all embedded in the social and political context of the society that shapes people's human, social, cultural, emotional and ecological resources. These multiple layers of factors and processes that shape people's health suggest that the 'care' of people's health must include appropriate action to create optimal conditions across all of them.

Figure1: Societal Determinants of People's Health

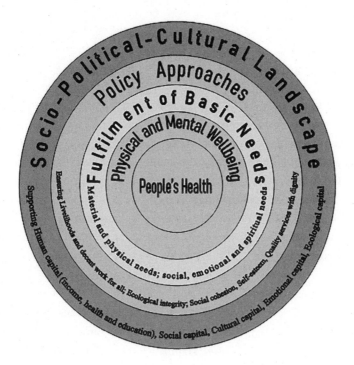

Ensuring a healthy India, therefore, requires a societal framing of health as one of the central objectives of social and economic development. Is it possible to dream that people's health and wellbeing will become a reference point in planning of all spheres, be it agriculture, industry, urban development, rural development, water and waste management, transport, energy, or any other, rather than achieving economic growth at the cost of people's health and wellbeing? Can policies and strategies factor in the negative impacts of development approaches on population health and also actively attempt to adopt approaches that impact health positively?

As a step towards this, the conception of health care must include three major levels of action, woven together in a holistic framework and as a societal endeavour:

1. The macro-level of social, economic and cultural conditions and policy approaches. These must be more conducive to health—distributive justice with dignity, an ethos of empathy and caring, collective thinking about health and ecological thinking.
2. An intermediate institutional level, with human health as a central object of all sectors. Health service systems must be developed in an optimal, cost-effective, people-centred systems design with individual health care embedded in efficient, empathetic and scientifically sound services, accessible to all.
3. Community-level action. People must come together for collective functioning and decision-making about the health of all members of society, along with empowerment of each individual for self-care and accessing appropriate health services when required.

The Sustainable Development Goals (SDGs) provide an international discourse that can facilitate adopting such an approach. The three pillars of sustainable development—environmental integrity, social justice and economic viability—are just as much relevant for healthy populations. SDG 3 is about 'ensuring health and wellbeing', but its strategy is narrowly focused on 'Universal Health Coverage with medical services financed through insurance'. WHO, UNICEF and the World Bank have reiterated the significance of a people-centred health-care approach,[7] yet do not seem to have broken out of the 'more of the same' approach. This is where rethinking the dominant approach and adopting transformative perspectives are required for sustainable health care that is empowering. Public health approaches that espouse more holistic perspectives can provide scientific inputs for such a re-centring of people's interests, giving direction and impetus towards health considerations in other spheres. However, moulding societal and policy thinking for reimagining health care towards sustainable and empowering systems will require concerted action and dreaming big!

Towards Health Services of Our Dreams: Realistic Visions

The healthiest of societies require health services for the prevention of ill health, its treatment and palliation with rehabilitation. Health service systems should thus be designed for the people they are meant for and their health-profile scenario. Technological effectiveness and safety, organizational and financial efficiency and quality of services are crucial features. The following diagram, Figure 2, illustrates the overarching frame and principal actions required. The two axes project the population increase by 2047, and the increasing population age with increasing life expectancy. The boxes depict the components of the system required to provide the services for acute and chronic health conditions of all. The arrows depict projected directions of future advances, one being most costly and least effective in increasing life expectancy, the other the least costly and most effective.

Figure 2: Framework for Strengthening the Indian Health Service System

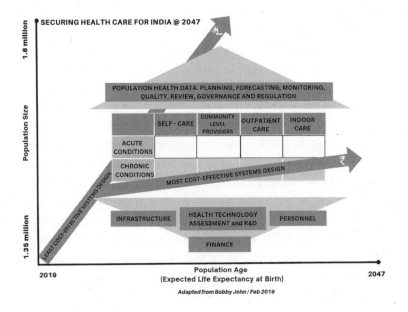

Adapted from Bobby John / Feb 2019

Designing such a health service system is a big challenge, as depicted in Figure 2. What should be the content of services, and how best can they be delivered? What approach would be optimally effective in improving people's health and wellbeing, and the most cost-effective, i.e., least expenditure and maximum health improvements, in comparison to the least cost-effective trajectory that is moving towards escalating medical costs with low health returns?

Acute and chronic illness requires a range of health care. From individuals in families and communities doing self-care, to formal and informal community health-care providers, to outdoor (OPD) and indoor institutional health services by formal service providers, all play decisive roles in health care even at present. Bringing them into a cooperative path is the most realistic and cost-effective design for a health-care system from this bottom-up perspective. Medical services will have to be seen as a social institution that is part of a wider range of preventive, curative, palliative and rehabilitative activities. Health-care services are wide and diverse, requiring various sectors and spheres to be brought into a coherent vision for the health of all. We will have to identify and design ways that are mutually reinforcing, empowering and sustainable at the societal level.

A holistic-health-systems approach that examines the historical experience of health services development and gives space to people's experience and knowledge, we think, is what will generate the most cost-effective trajectory. It will be most easily operationalized if the government agencies and the community come together to play a leading role in health care. All health-care providers, including the private sector, would have to be socialized according to the needs of a people-centred vision of health. Dependence on the private sector as the leader in the sector can only be a recipe for the least cost-effective trajectory of Figure 2, characterized by high costs of health care to society and low returns. It will over-medicalize health care, and lead to greater dependence on medical technology and specialist-led services, with loss of self-care and community-level providers.

The most cost-effective trajectory may seem like an unrealistic dream at this juncture, where a highly commercialized health service system seems to have got accepted as the norm. However, it needs to be remembered that societies have, at various periods of time including the present, provided treatment services as an altruistic or a philanthropic or state-supported free service for the ill and suffering. It is only in the past four decades of this neo-liberal era that we have witnessed a policy-supported, pervasive commercialization and corporatization of medical services at unaffordable levels.

The structure of the population and changing trends by age, gender and regional distribution provide the first layer of information for planning. Data gathering and surveillance systems about health and disease become crucial in this regard. People's health-related behaviours and practices form the second and the available health-care resources the third data sets that are required.

A 'continuum of care', then, has to be ensured by the health service system, from self-care capacities to community-level providers and professional medical care through outdoor and indoor institutional services, catering to varied needs at appropriate levels. Infrastructure, personnel, technologies, financing and governance have to be strengthened with a comprehensive vision. Monitoring and regulation for equity and quality assurance are important components for governance of the health services.

Thus, the divides and prioritization between health service and non-health service inputs, public and private formal services, conventional modern and other/traditional knowledges, the formal and informal health care, and layperson and experts, need to be addressed. These are the various grids that need to be kept in mind as we imagine the health system and its strengthening, to generate dialogue across the divides for a democratic health care system. *A democratic health care system means one that is inclusive, comprehensive, effective, context-sensitive, plural, sustainable and empowering.*

Essays in This Volume

This volume, we hope, will provide some understanding and answers to resolve the dilemmas and debates in contemporary health systems development. The first six essays will lay out the wider landscape of health care and a vision for creating a healthful society while the next seven will focus on innovations for health services development.

The first essay lays out the demographic and disease profile of the Indian population for the coming decades. The second moves to a description of the social determinants of health and how to deal with them through a 'Health in All Policies' approach, also arguing for people's committees to ensure grounded inputs and implementation. The third essay argues for bringing the idea of complexity back into public health planning. Drawing out a history of complex planning efforts, it shows how, over the years, this nuanced understanding about what shapes health and health problems and how to deal with them has reduced, leading to failures of policy and programme implementation in independent India. It proposes resurrecting the complex planning vision of the Nehru–Mahalanobis imagination along with addressing the structural barriers to equality, dignity and human rights of all, to realize the dream of building public health in India. Adding to the complexity of the health-care landscape, the fourth essay draws attention to the continuum of multiple traditions of knowledge that survive as live sources of understanding human health, health problems and their preventive practices and treatment solutions. Addressing this cultural plurality, the essay demonstrates with strong examples the complementarity of the modern/Western/ European knowledge system (as it is variously called) and that of the earlier/traditional/indigenous/Southern/Eastern health sciences and practices. Thereby, it argues for building 'integrative health sciences' by drawing on their complementarity and the strengths of each for a health science of the twenty-first century. The fifth essay draws upon learnings from civil society-led rural health-care initiatives. It brings the humane element of health-care providers to the fore, illustrating innovations in primary health care that have been implemented successfully across the country through people-centred initiatives. It explains how they provide directions for inclusive health care of the future, including learnings that can be implemented for re-orienting public services. The sixth essay deals with the need for planning with endogenous perspectives to design policies and services suited to context. It analyses the specific case of Acute Encephalitis Syndrome child deaths in Gorakhpur to highlight the gaps in approaches used to address public health problems. Examples of urban planning and of health systems design demonstrate the need for rethinking how we plan our systems in much more context-suited ways. It proposes that this requires bottom-up approaches to research and planning, especially inclusive of perspectives of the marginalized sections. The role of people's informal arrangements, perceptions, and handling of systemic challenges in these domains is highlighted as a resource for systems development.

The next seven essays examine innovative approaches for most cost-effective systems design, addressing the many dimensions of health services development. The first essay among them, i.e., the seventh essay after this introductory essay, reflects on the most critical problem the public health services in India are presently facing—of adequate human resources for health care. It traces the historical development of health services in the country to identify how we have ended up in such a crisis, focusing on the conundrum of ensuring adequate and appropriate health-care professionals. It recommends several key measures to remedy the number and quality of health human resources in relation to people's needs and to meet the demands of Universal Health Care.

The eighth essay presents a 'new' health-care paradigm in that it deals with the present fragmentation of services by primary, secondary and tertiary institutions and presents a framework for patient-centred services from womb to tomb, with appropriate forward and backward referral pathways between the three levels of institutions. While discussing the continuum of care in relation to several health problems areas, it illustrates the integrated health-care pathways through management of chronic kidney disease patients.

The ninth essay draws lessons for a futuristic vision of secondary and tertiary hospitals from the experience of several hospitals being run in the non-profit sector. The infrastructural, clinical and operational models are generalizable for all health services to emulate, whether in the government, private or non-profit sector. This re-visioning of hospitals, from the giant-size, glass-and-marble and 'latest-technology' ideal of the present corporate hospitals, to more rational, cost-effective institutions sensitive to local socio-cultural and ecological contexts, architecturally and functionally, is the only way that adequate hospital care can be provided to all, with good quality and in a sustainable way. Otherwise they are too capital intensive without added service quality or health outcomes. The tenth essay spells out the urgency for community-based mental health care along with strengthening of psychiatric services. It also argues for non-medical community-based preventive mental wellbeing strategies. Finding hope in several recent developments in the country in relation to mental health laws and learnings from civil society initiatives, it highlights the need to correct previous approaches by integrating physical and mental health care services, adopting a human-rights lens, and addressing the physical and social causation of mental illnesses.

The eleventh essay deals with ways of regulating and socializing the private health services sector for public good. This is critical to enhance the private health sector's accountability and generate trust. Drawing from the COVID pandemic measures where public systems drew upon private hospitals for handling the public health crisis, it provides a coherent vision for how the private service system can be better utilized and mobilized to provide better outcomes for the Indian people. It suggests a three-pronged mechanism of social regulation of the health sector combining state regulation, multi-stakeholder accountability and self-regulation. The twelfth essay gives extremely valuable new insights into the governance and research management issues at the highest leadership level of the central Ministry of Health and Family Welfare. It is decisions at these levels that shape the formal structure, content and functional capacities of the health-care system in the country. Examining the persistent structural contestations within the health governance institutions in the country, it recommends restructuring of governance and knowledge architecture and functioning in ways that are also essential to bring about the innovations recommended in the other chapters. It focuses on the persistent contestations in the health administration between the Centre and the states and the administrator-technical knowledge leadership. It also includes an analysis of the potential benefits and prevailing challenges of the use of Information Technologies in health governance.

The last essay in the volume portrays creative health systems innovations made by the young central Indian state of Chhattisgarh. It very succinctly demonstrates the possibility of implementation of the kind of public policy orientation and innovations advocated for in the other papers. It demonstrates the potential of a public and civil society/citizens partnership in evolving an effective health-care system through real-life policymaking in the twenty-first century. It also demonstrates the significance of the freedom that the states can constitutionally exercise in response to their diverse contexts, and the kind of eco-system that generates continuous innovations for strengthening the health-care system.

Thus, as readers go through the volume, they will find that all essays present practical solutions with an explanation of the principles on which these are based. These solutions will be found feasible for giving shape to the vision of a public-community-partnership based system, and can be adopted by the private sector as win-win solutions. The volume does not include a specific essay on financing health care, but its underlying framework, as depicted in Figures 1 and 2, is that the relationship of economic and social development planning with health care is not about financing medical and health services alone, it is about gearing our socio-economic development efforts towards a healthy environment, human health and wellbeing, and adopting the most cost-effective health care systems design. If such a vision guides political decision-making, it will include providing more resources to caring for those suffering ill-health than the public budget has given so far. Further, several essays point to financing issues. Innovations in systems design presented across the essays and the rational and appropriate use of health technologies will keep funding requirements for the Indian health service system cost-effective and societally affordable.

The volume provides innovative ideas for various elements of what is needed to build a 'people-centred health-care system'. Across essays, these add up to a holistic vision that vastly differs from the prevalent doctor- and hospital-centered imagination of health care that medical insurance attempts to make seem affordable while real costs escalate. This holistic vision, based on the reality of everyday lives of people and their perceptions and aspirations, as well as those of the health-care service providers, is not only doable because all the ideas emerge from experience of their practice, but also desirable as leading to a win-win situation for all providers and users of services. However, its implementation depends on the revitalization of public institutions, with organic linkages to the agency of the people they are meant to serve. It requires strong political will, democratic governance and public vigilance to make the shift to such a vision of health care.

This vision contributes to the spirit of a democratic society. Such a health-care system will be integral to building the India of our dreams.

We had the benefit of the spade work done towards this volume at Samruddha Bharat Foundation earlier by Dr Bobby John. We acknowledge this gratefully, but we take responsibility for the shape the volume has finally taken.

India's Population Structure and Health Priorities of the Twenty-First Century

Purushottam M. Kulkarni and Rajib Dasgupta

Introduction

As India embarked on the path of planned development post-Independence, rapid population growth was one of the major issues to be confronted. The rise in the rate of growth was brought about by a decline in mortality—in itself a welcome development. As a further decline in mortality was desired and expected, the population growth rate was bound to rise unless there was a corresponding fall in fertility. The persistence of high fertility and, consequently, high population growth caused concern to the planners. However, by the 1990s, evidence began to emerge that fertility had declined in most parts of the country.

Several factors contributed to the fall in fertility.[1] Decline in infant and child mortality meant that most newborns survived to adulthood, thus obviating the need to have many children to ensure that at least a few would survive. Socioeconomic changes like the monetization of the economy raised aspirations and couples found it in their interest to have fewer children so that they could spend more on their development, especially education—the classical quantity-quality trade-off. Mass media and door-to-door canvassing by grassroots-level workers and easy availability of contraceptives, free of cost, under the family planning programme promoted the small family norm.

Clearly, the classical demographic transition, in which there is a decline in mortality followed by a downward curve in fertility, has been in progress in India for quite some time. How will this impact India's population growth and structure in the foreseeable future? This essay discusses India's population prospects in the twenty-first century and its implications for health and health-care needs.

Population Prospects in the Twenty-First Century

The 2001 census enumerated India's population at 103 crore, that is, over one billion. At the same time, it showed a small decline in the pace of population growth,[2] with the annual rate falling marginally below the 2 per cent mark. But this change in trend was hardly given any attention; the crossing of the billion-mark dominated public discourse. However, ten years later, when the 2011 census enumerated the population at 121 crore, it was seen that the annual growth rate had fallen well below 2 per cent. A downward trend had clearly begun in the trajectory of the growth rate. Further, the Total Fertility Rate (TFR), the average number of births per woman over her lifetime if she survives through the reproductive span, fell to 2.18 in 2017.[3] Given the mortality level at the time, India can be said to have reached the commonly sought low 'replacement level' fertility, thus completing the demographic transition.

But achieving replacement level fertility does not immediately stop population growth. The momentum of population growth and anticipated decline in mortality means the population will grow for some more time. India's population will, therefore, continue to increase for a while, though at a slower pace, before declining due to the predicted fall in fertility below the replacement level. According to the latest projections by the United Nations Population Division, U.N. World Population Prospects, 2022 (UNWPP-2022), India's population will reach a peak of 170 crore by 2064 and decline thereafter to about 153 crore by the end of the century (the projections of the Medium variant of the UNWPP are used here as this variant is generally accepted as the most likely).[4] An independent projection, the 'reference' variant in a recent paper in the *Lancet* shows a peak of 161 crore for India by 2048, lower than that in the UN Medium variant, and a relatively sharper decline after that to 109 crore by 2100.[5] Figure 1 depicts the population trajectories as per these projections.

While the assumptions made in alternate projections are debatable, it is now amply clear that India has reached low replacement fertility and further decline in fertility is imminent. Population growth in India, therefore, will cease sometime around the middle of the century and population size will begin to decline

Figure 1: Projected population (in crore), India, 2020 to 2100, UNWPP-2022 Medium variant and *Lancet* 2020 paper, 'Reference' variant.

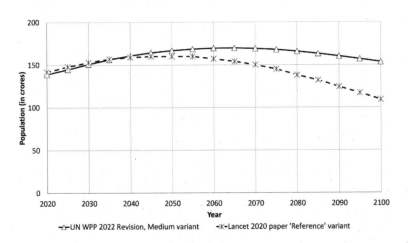

slowly. Both the projections cited show a peak between 161 and 170 crore, a growth of less than 50 crore, that is, about 40 per cent over the 2011 census population. Thus, the dread of population explosion, commonly expressed during the second half of the twentieth century, is no longer a concern. The goal of 'population control', stated often in public discourses, can be said to have been achieved.

Age Structure Set to Change Radically

Through the century, however, India's population will undergo major structural changes. Broadly, it will age. With a decline in fertility, the annual number of births will decrease over time after 2020. As a result, the young population, of ages below fifteen years, will decline in size and share. The working-age population—fifteen to sixty-four years—will rise for some time. Besides, as childhood mortality has declined and is projected to fall further, most of the birth cohorts will survive longer. A notable consequence, frequently mentioned in discussions on development in recent years, is the demographic dividend this rise in share of working-age population will yield. But this will be a passing phase, called the 'window of demographic opportunity'. The bulge in the middle-age share of the population will gradually move upwards and pass on to the older ages, causing a phenomenal rise in the share of elderly population. This rise is projected to continue throughout the century. In 2011, less than 6 per cent of India's population was of ages sixty-five and above,[6] but according to the 'Medium' fertility variant of the UNWPP-2022, the share of the population above the age of sixty-five is projected to rise to 15 per cent by 2050 and 30 per cent by 2100.[7] The rise in the share of the very old, above eighty years of age, will be relatively steeper, from less than 1 per cent in 2011 to close to 3 per cent by 2050 and 12 per cent by 2100. On the other hand, the share of the young population, below the age of fifteen, which was 31 per cent in 2011, is projected to fall to 18 per cent by 2050 and further to 14 per cent by 2100. The share of the working-age population is projected to rise from 64 per cent in 2011 to a peak of 69 per cent in the late 2030s and then gradually decline. This means that the dependency ratio, the proportion of population outside working ages to the working-age population (15–64 years), will fall from 57 per cent in 2011 to a low of 45 per cent in the late 2030s but begin to rise after 2040 and is expected to be over 50 per cent by 2060 and over 75 per cent by 2100.

The standard graphical depiction of the population structure is called a 'population pyramid' since in the past the shape of the graph resembled a pyramid, with a heavy bottom (representing the young ages) gradually becoming thinner as one moves upwards in age. This will no longer be the case. Soon, India's population pyramid will not look like a pyramid but rather like a barrel with some unevenness (the pyramids for 2011, 2050 and 2100 are shown in Figure 2).[8]

Socioeconomic and Spatial Variations in Transition

The empirical evidence clearly shows that declines in mortality and fertility have occurred in all sections of India's population, cutting across social categories and economic classes and in rural as well as urban areas. Though socioeconomic differentials in levels of fertility and mortality do exist, these have been narrowing over time and the future paths for all sections are quite similar. There are, no doubt, conspicuous differences in the initiation and timing of the demographic transition among regions of India, and consequently the changes in the age structure will also differ spatially. Over half of the large states have already reached replacement level fertility and their populations are expected to peak in the next two or three decades and then experience decline. But fertility decline has occurred in all regions of the country and given the recent trends, replacement level is expected to be achieved in the foreseeable future in the remaining states as well.

Since the states lagging in the transition will reach the peak later (but well before the end of this century), population ageing will be delayed. This spells huge regional imbalances in future population growth and pressures for inter-state migration.

Figure 2: Population Pyramids, India, 2011 Census and 2050 and 2100 Projected (UNWPP-2022 Revision, Medium variant), Population in Millions

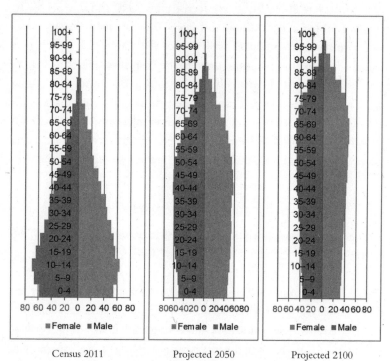

Census 2011	Projected 2050	Projected 2100

Source: The 2011 pyramid is constructed from the age-sex distribution of the 2011 census and the 2050 and 2100 pyramids from the projected age-sex distributions given in the Medium variant of UNWPP-2022

Implications for Health Needs

During the last century, the principal population-related issue for India was the enormous growth, with population size more than quadrupling through the century. However, in the present century, changes in the age structure, rather than growth, will be the main aspect of population that will figure in policies and plans. This has a bearing on health needs and services. The burden of disease is heavily influenced by the age-sex structure in addition to epidemiologic conditions. It is well recognized that prevalence of specific morbidities varies by age. As population ages, there will be greater requirement for the treatment of non-communicable, degenerative and lifestyle diseases. Many among the very old also need palliative care. At the same time, pregnancy, delivery and neonatal care also need to be strengthened; though early childhood and maternal mortality rates have declined significantly in India, the present levels are still unacceptably high. Nutritional intakes also differ by age as does the need for preventive care. Clearly, the anticipated change in the age structure will have major implications for health needs and planning for health services.

The Changing Epidemiology of Diseases

Urbanization, mechanization and globalization have led to unprecedented changes in lifestyle, including physical activity and food habits, such as shifts away from traditional diets.[9] India is undergoing a major *epidemiological transition*, marked by a shift in disease patterns. This is marked by a substantial decline in mortality on account of communicable, maternal, neonatal and nutritional diseases (CMNNDs) and increase in non-communicable diseases (NCDs) and injuries to the overall disease burden.

Epidemiological transition is a relatively broad-brush concept, with further nuances. *Epidemiological acceleration* signifies an epidemiological transition in developing countries and transition economies in the absence of the improvements in social and economic wellbeing experienced in advanced economies. *Epidemiological polarization* refers to the growing increase in health inequalities between countries, regions and social groups; it is the most vulnerable populations that experience excess morbidity and mortality from a variety of causes.[10] The poorest experience the highest death rates owing to both pre-transitional diseases, including infections and nutritional disorders, and rising NCDs.[11] The phenomenon was demonstrated in the context of Kerala about a decade ago.[12] Ominously, the protracted polarization model is accelerated with rapid urbanization.[13] Analysis of the Study on Global Ageing and Adult Health suggests that while several NCDs were concentrated among the lower socio-economic groups, self-reported cases were higher among higher socio-economic groups.[14] The chronic diseases burden in India can be attributed to an interaction of individual behaviours and social environments (Figure 3).[15]

Figure 3: Contribution of major disease groups to total Disability Adjusted Life Years (DALYs) in India, 1990 and 2016

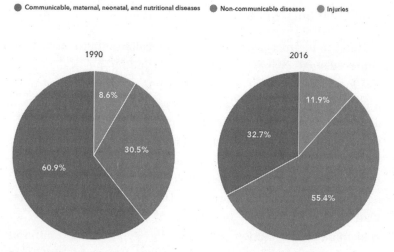

Source: India: Health of the Nation's States: the India State-Level Disease Burden Initiative

While the global burden of diseases is expressed in terms of DALYs (Disability Adjusted Life Years), a more sensitive measure is the *epidemiological transition ratio* (ETR). It is the ratio of DALYs caused by communicable, maternal, neonatal and nutritional diseases versus those caused by non-communicable diseases and injuries. The lower the ratio, the greater the contribution of NCDs and injuries to a state's overall disease burden. Most states had ratios more than one in 1990; by 2016, all states had ratios less than one—underscoring the contribution of NCDs and injuries to premature death and disability (Figure 4). The states with the highest ETR include Kerala (0.16), Goa, Tamil Nadu, Punjab and Himachal Pradesh. States with high ETR are Bihar (0.74), Jharkhand, Uttar Pradesh, Rajasthan, Chhattisgarh and Madhya Pradesh.

Figure 4: Epidemiological transition ratios of the states of India, 2016

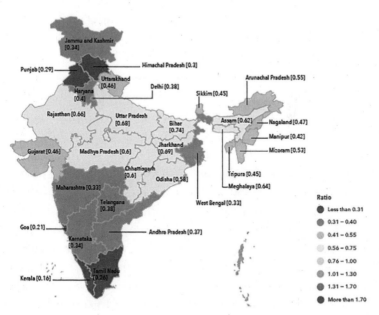

Source: India: Health of the Nation's States: The India State-Level Disease Burden Initiative

These issues point to a somewhat unique health policy and health service requirements of each state, not just at present but in their planning for the next several decades, in sync with demographic transition. The high ETR states are among the Empowered Action Group (EAG) states that receive special focus under the National Health Mission (NHM).

The Shift Towards the Urban

While India continues to be primarily rural in many states and districts, the country has been urbanizing; an estimated half of the population shall be urban in the coming decade or so. However, the urbanization is undirected, random and opportunistic—shaped more by pressures than policies. Of particular concern are the fast-expanding peri-urban areas and populations, for which there are neither estimates nor policies. The urban population, 377 million as per the 2011 Census, recorded a decadal increase of 91 million in the last decade (2001–11). The UN World Urbanization Prospects report estimates that more than two-thirds of the world will live in urban areas by 2050; India's urban share is to be 53 per cent.[16]

Urban living is generally associated with advantages in economic opportunity, living standards and access to services. Though organization of and access to health and other basic municipal services may often be easier, there can be significant issues of inclusion and exclusion.[17] The 'urbanization of poverty' thesis proposes that cities entrench inequalities by ghettoizing poverty and 'enclaving' affluence in close and stark proximity.[18] A UN projection forecasted that global urban share of poverty will reach 40 per cent in 2020 when the urban share of the population is projected to reach 52 per cent.[19] The urban share of the total number of poor was projected to reach 50 per cent by 2035, when the urban population share is expected to be 61 per cent.[20]

The urban poor pay disproportionately higher prices and costs for urban infrastructure and services, a phenomenon characterized as 'informal survivalism'.[21] This connects to serious concerns about increasing disparities in the health condition of the populations within the same city. Data from rounds of the National Family Health Surveys consistently records that the urban poor experience worse health outcomes in comparison to the urban non-poor and residents of rural areas; the urban poor have higher under-five mortality, underweight population and disproportionate vulnerability to respiratory and vector-borne diseases as well as non-communicable diseases such as diabetes, hypertension and mental distress in comparison to rural populations. Further, they are highly susceptible to communicable and chronic epidemics due to the degraded nature of their living and working environment. The National Health Profile 2019 indicates that several communicable diseases have a high case fatality rate (above 2 per cent): Rabies (100 per cent), Japanese Encephalitis (11 per cent), H1N1 Influenza (7 per cent), Acute Encephalitis Syndrome (6 per cent), Encephalitis (5 per cent), Meningococcal Meningitis (4 per cent) and Diphtheria (2 per cent).[22]

Urban Vulnerabilities Will Be the New Challenge

The National Urban Health Mission (NUHM) has framed urban vulnerability across three axes: residential or habitat-based vulnerability, social vulnerability (e.g., female-headed households and minor-headed households or those based on caste, religion and state or linguistic identities) and occupational vulnerability (e.g., urban persons/households without access to social security and susceptible to significant periods of unemployment).

Recent global reports point to roadmaps for action. The WHO Commission on Social Determinants of Health (CSDH) called for promoting health equity between rural and urban areas.[23, 24] A *Lancet* editorial argued for prioritizing and equitably addressing urban health in the post-MDG era through a three-pronged approach: governments committing to improving urban health by prioritizing equitable access and adapted delivery of health and related services to the urban poor and non-legal residents; pursuing Sustainable Development Goal (SDG) 11 including increased investment in safe, accessible public transportation, improving air and water quality for all and especially for the poor, and the use of modern low-emission and renewable energy sources for cooking and heating in homes; and, focusing on health in the design of these smaller cities.[25]

In Summary

India has now reached replacement-level fertility and is set to enter a phase of sub-replacement fertility and thus, the fears of population explosion have faded out. But demographic processes entail that the age structure will undergo major changes and the population is expected to age. At present, the age distribution of the Indian population (and of populations in most of the developing world) is vastly different from that of the developed world. This has been the case for quite some time, as the demographic transition began quite early in the developed world. In 2020, only 16 per cent of the population in the developed world was younger than fifteen while 19 per cent was aged sixty-five or higher. Thus, ageing has been in progress in most of the developed world and the health services in these countries are already attuned to cater to the large elderly population. Given that change in the age structure is necessarily gradual, health services can adapt over time to accommodate it. Besides, much can be learned from the experience of the developed world.

As evidence builds up, the understanding of the challenges of an ageing and urban population will become more refined. Communicable diseases shall remain important among children and in adults, as TB, malaria and HIV continue to be endemic notwithstanding their elimination targets, and vector-borne diseases keep resurfacing in urban and peri-urban avatars. The COVID-19 pandemic points to additional challenges from a range of zoonoses. NCDs, injuries and disabilities shall, however, continue to dominate the epidemiological discourse. Expanding urban and peri-urban populations and increasing rural–urban human movements will lead to both dissemination of infections and lifestyles. Health policies and health services shall need to reckon with these rapid changes in demographic and location contexts. Addressing emerging health inequalities and inequities in India as a moral imperative should not only be our dream, but a reality too.

Ensuring Health for All, in All Policies

K. Srinath Reddy

Why Health?

Health has both intrinsic and instrumental value for any human being. The intrinsic value comes from feeling fit, having a sense of wellbeing and the ability for self-care, capability to participate in pleasant social interactions and sports as one chooses to, enjoy loving relationships, have sex and rear children as desired. The instrumental value comes from opportunities provided by good health to access education, employment, earn good income, gain financial security, participate in competitive sports or performing arts and contribute to societal development. Health is, therefore, rightly regarded by many as a human right that must be protected and promoted. Such a view positions health in the framework of social justice and calls on all of society to recognize and respect this right.[1, 2]

Besides what an individual gains from good health, society too gains from the health of its citizens. The increased productivity of healthy workers contributes to economic growth. When a country is not burdened by debilitating physical illnesses which impose high health and economic costs or challenged by a high level of mental health disruptions among its people, it can enjoy social harmony. Epidemics can derail economic activity. Even non-infectious diseases like cardiovascular diseases, diabetes and cancers can create unstable labour and consumer markets by endangering a productive workforce, diverting personal and family savings to high-cost health care and subtracting spending power for other preferred purchases.

Health across the Life Course

Challenges to health vary across life, in diversity and intensity. Infectious and nutritional disorders can occur anytime but are especially frequent at both extremes of life, with still evolving immunity in young children and declining immunity in the elderly. Adolescence has its own challenges, from onset of addictive and other at-risk behaviours to stress-related mental health challenges. Pregnancy and childbirth pose dangers to women whose health may have already been adversely affected by undernutrition and anaemia carried from childhood through adolescence. Through the decades of adulthood, risks of non-communicable diseases (NCDs) rise, resulting in increasing burdens of cardiovascular, renal and respiratory diseases, diabetes and cancers. Health services, thus, must be provided as appropriate to the needs of health at each stage of life.

Further, the health of any individual must be seen to commence in the womb of the mother where the body is genetically configured, anatomically structured and physiologically programmed. Health at every subsequent stage of life is influenced by the health experience—positive or negative—in the preceding stage.

Determinants of Health

Several social, economic, environmental and commercial determinants of health influence beliefs and behaviours to impact biological processes within the human body, to promote or imperil physical and mental health. These determinants operate at both population and individual levels and frequently interact with each other to influence health across the life course.[3]

While these determinants are often grouped in different clusters, all of them are determined by the political processes that organize and govern society. Thus, the political economy of health cannot be separated from the commercial determinants, nor can the environmental determinants be addressed without regulating economic activities that impact the environment. It is the weave of these many determinants that scripts the health of populations and steers the health of individuals across their life course. The WHO Commission on Social Determinants of Health has drawn the attention of the global health community and policymakers to the imperative of bridging the gaps through greater attention to health in all policies so that the 'causes of causes' can be addressed.[4]

Economic Determinants

The economic status of countries and the level of inequality within them influence health in many ways. The economic growth of a country and the health of its population have a bidirectional relationship, with material conditions affecting the health of the population which in turn affects economic activity and its productivity. The Preston curve illustrates how life expectancy at birth correlates positively to per capita GDP till a plateauing effect occurs at higher levels.[5] Distributional equity also helps countries achieve higher gains in health for any rise in per capita GDP, with countries with higher levels of equity presenting better population-level health and other social indicators than countries in a comparable income category but with higher levels of inequity.[6] Countries too cannot spend on creating efficient and equitable health systems if their health budgets are insufficient due to debt-ridden economies which suffer slow growth. The stark differences between rich countries and all others in being able to quickly access and administer vaccines against COVID-19 is a striking reminder of the role economic differences among countries play in global health.[7]

At the individual level, poverty and ill health too have a bidirectional relationship, with one precipitating or perpetuating the other. From the ability to live in safe housing and being able to buy nutritious foods to accessing health information and affording appropriate health care, economic factors significantly impinge on an individual's health.

Education

Education positively influences health at the individual level.[8] The level of formal education, which has been most studied in this regard, shows positive correlation. Health and nutrition literacy additionally foster healthier habits and guide appropriate health-seeking behaviours. Education opens the path for higher income-generating occupations, lowering the risk of poverty and enabling affordable health care. Gender sensitivity and equity are expected but not always realized benefits of education. However, women's education, empowerment and employment in income-earning occupations have been consistently associated with better health status of families, states and countries.[9] Good education also reduces information asymmetry and addresses the imbalance of decision-making power that separates the health-care provider from the person accessing health services.

Poverty, gender, race, religion, caste and conflict pose barriers to education and prevent economically or socially disadvantaged sections of society from accessing formal and non-formal knowledge that promotes health. Both formal and non-formal modes of learning must be easily accessible to all if health has to benefit from people's awareness of what protects and what harms and how health services have to be availed.

Nutrition

A vital determinant of health, nutrition supports growth, enables renewal of cells and tissues, promotes immunity, produces hormones and provides energy for our daily activities. It provides the chemistry for our life by supplying the building blocks of our biology.

Malnutrition, which poses many threats to health, is a multi-faceted problem. Conventionally, it has been compartmentalized into undernutrition, overnutrition and micro-nutrient deficiencies. This is an erroneous over-simplification. All of these can overlap in the same individual at different stages of life or even exist at the same time in an individual. Undernutrition during pregnancy or early childhood can lead to higher levels of body fat (adiposity) and less lean muscle in later childhood and adulthood, resulting in 'metabolic obesity' with many adverse health effects. An overweight or obese individual may have micronutrient deficiencies and often has a diet low in fruit, vegetables, dietary fibre and healthier fats. Healthy nutrition depends on dietary diversity, which provides adequate energy (calories) while ensuring an appropriate mix of nutrients in right quantities and proportions.[10]

Agriculture and Food Systems

Provision of nutritionally rich diets to the entire population, at affordable prices, is the function of agriculture and food systems. Dietary diversity depends on crop diversity, while the nutrient quality of the crops depends on the type of soil, type and quantity of chemicals used as fertilizers or pesticides, the adequacy of irrigation and, increasingly, climate change. Food supply depends on the yield, which varies according to soil, seed, irrigation and climate; it is also impacted by post-harvest losses that are dependent on socio-economically influenced systems of storage, food safety and transport. These factors affect health by determining the quantity of food available to the population through domestic national production. Besides these, transnational trade alters the dynamics of food supply. Commercial considerations in agricultural systems result in preference for cash crops (such as tobacco), in preference to nutrient-rich crops. Mono-cropping of commercially preferred plants has also adversely affected crop diversity.[11]

It is in the areas of processing, pricing, marketing and promotion of food products that health is greatly undermined by commercial determinants. Ultra-processed foods, with high levels of salt, sugar and trans-fats, are also often devoid of fibre and essential nutrients.[12] Energy-dense but nutrient-poor foods and beverages are aggressively marketed and promoted through many types of advertising. Apart from being intrinsically harmful to health, they also displace healthy food products from the diet. Food prices also limit the ability of the poor from accessing healthier options like fruit, vegetables and edible oils of desirable quality. Food price fluctuations, caused by economic downturns in national economies or disruption of global supply chains, can be catastrophic to the poor.[13] Food waste is an increasing contributor to malnutrition even when production is adequate.[14]

Urban Design and Transport

Apart from diet, a cardinal and complementary component of health is physical activity, which sets the demand for nutrients and helps us to utilize them efficiently. Low muscle mass, resulting from low, inadequate or inappropriate diets, can limit an individual's capacity for physical activity. However, even those who wish to be physically active are impeded by urban design and transport systems which limit human mobility. Without safe pedestrian pathways and protected cycling lanes, unplanned urban growth prevents physically active commuting. Availability of mass public transport systems will enable people to walk to their destinations at both ends of the commute, rather than depend on cars or two-wheelers to carry them from doorstep to doorstep.[15] Traffic safety is another area of urban planning and governance that needs attention to reduce the growing burden of road accidents which kill or maim many.

The built environment of cities also influences the aptitude and ability of people to be physically active. Large, open green and brown spaces, which permit safe and pleasurable physical activity, are needed in urban areas but are fast shrinking or disappearing due to unplanned or commercially motivated construction. Parks, playgrounds and open-air gyms are becoming endangered in many areas as urban growth sacrifices open spaces for closed buildings. Large-scale migration from rural areas and urban poverty create overcrowded slums that carry many health hazards.

Water and Sanitation

The importance of clean water and sanitation in preventing myriad infectious diseases has been well-recognized for centuries. Indeed, the foundations of modern public health were laid when water and sanitation services were improved to counter killer diseases like cholera and typhoid. Vector-borne diseases too, like malaria, dengue and chikungunya, thrive in the absence of clean water and sanitation.

Sanitary conditions in urban slums are especially distressing.[16] Overcrowding, water shortages and irregular collection and disposal of garbage pose several health hazards. Inadequate health services compound the problem. Even in rural areas, poor sanitation and non-availability of potable water pose serious challenges to health. Policies that are directed at rural and urban development must be especially attentive to these basic needs.

Environment

From air pollution to global warming, the physical environment is becoming a major threat to health instead of being a supportive source. This inimical transformation is almost entirely anthropogenic—a result of misguided developmental priorities. Emissions, construction dust and use of biomass fuels have raised air pollution to levels that cause high burdens of cardiovascular, respiratory, reproductive and metabolic disorders as well as cancer.[17]

Extensive deforestation, steeply rising industrial and vehicular emissions and industrial-scale animal breeding for meat consumption have accelerated climate change. Climate change harms health through heat effects, extreme weather events, vector- and water-borne infections, cardiovascular diseases, mental health disorders and several other health hazards.[18] Food systems are adversely affected as production of both staples and non-staples is adversely affected. The nutrient quality of staples is impacted, with a consequent rise in the number of people suffering from deficiency of zinc, iron and protein. Fruit and vegetable production and preservation is affected by heat. Warming of sea water will endanger marine fish and rising sea waters will inundate farms and damage cultivation of crops in coastal areas.

Gender

While biological determinants like the strength of the immune system and higher levels of HDL cholesterol favour women's health and facilitate higher life expectancy in comparison to males, the adverse impact of many social determinants undermines women's health and threatens the lives and wellbeing of many women across the world. Lower economic status, reduced educational and employment opportunities, gender-based discrimination and violence, neglected nutritional needs and lower access to health care are factors which contribute to poor health and wellbeing among women.[19]

Patriarchal attitudes in society over several generations and feudal social structures and cultural practices that force girls into early marriage are among the adverse factors that undermine women's health. Lack of financial independence leads to denied or delayed health care. Exposure to indoor air pollution, when subjected to burning biomass fumes in the kitchen, drudgery of fetching water from long distances, lack of access to sanitary supplies and contraception are among the many challenges that women face.[20] When gender-based discrimination is superimposed on discrimination due to caste, religion, ethnicity or language, the impact on health is even more adverse.

Conflict, Violence and Social Instability

Both physical and mental health can be greatly endangered by conflicts in society, especially if they are violent. While wars are an extreme form of attack on health, even low-intensity conflicts, if long-drawn, can disrupt the economic, physical and mental wellbeing of people and disrupt health systems. Forced migration, due to war, ethnic cleansing or climate-related emergencies, is an increasing phenomenon in the twenty-first century, and has had demonstrated adverse effects on health.[21, 22]

Social instability and discrimination is the lived reality of many minority groups and has adverse effects on their mental and physical health. Not infrequently, they are also subjected to physical violence which inflicts serious damage on health.

Health in All Policies

Given the impact that political, economic, social, environmental and commercial determinants have on the health of populations and individuals, they need to be shaped to positively influence health. This requires policy instruments that can steer change at the population level, not merely behavioural interventions that focus on changing knowledge, attitude and practice at the individual level.

Policy interventions are non-personal but have a population-wide impact, if well-conceived and effectively implemented.[23]

They are often cost-saving and can involve fiscal instruments which provide revenue that can be used for health promotion and delivery of universal health care. They also have inter-generational benefits, by creating food systems, urban designs and pollution control mechanisms which continue to provide health benefits in the future.

Tobacco control is an area where policy instruments have been effectively used. Raising taxes on tobacco products increases their price and curbs consumption, especially among the vulnerable groups with low disposable incomes. Bans on advertising, promotion and sponsorship of tobacco products has reduced the ability of the industry to entice and entrap new customers into experimentation with the highly addictive nicotine-delivery systems. Prominent pictorial health warnings on tobacco product packs, mandated by law, convey information on the health hazards of tobacco use, which the tobacco industry is eager to hide. A ban on smoking in public places and indoor workplaces protects many from the dangers of second-hand smoke.[24]

The food industry too needs to be regulated through policies which mandate the reduction of unhealthy ingredients in ultra-processed foods. Fiscal interventions, through a judicious mix of taxes and subsidies, can make unhealthy food products costlier and healthier products more affordable. Advertising restrictions are needed too, to control the promotion of 'junk' foods and sugary drinks. Food labels can help guide consumer choice by differentiating healthier products from those which are likely to harm health.[25, 26]

Climate change needs a concerted response across many sectors, from energy alternatives to fossil fuels, to reversing the loss of green cover from deforestation, reducing methane emissions from livestock and deep decarbonization strategies.[27]

Aligning policies in other sectors to health policy objectives is not easy. Those sectors act according to their priorities and may view public health objectives as secondary or even conflicting with their goals. Promoting commercial crops and food products which do not meet nutrient needs may be defended on their contribution to economic growth. Similarly, curbs on fossil fuels may be resisted by advancing arguments that there is a development lag which needs to be bridged first. An alibi often offered for policymaker inaction is that national data is sparse and international data is not contextually relevant. Commercial interests often resist policy interventions by raising the flag of 'individual choice'. However, that choice is seldom free. It is often conditioned by aggressive marketing and promotion of unhealthy products by the industry. It is also conditioned by industry-manipulated peer pressure. Even if people are fully aware of the right health information, their choice may be constrained by economic circumstances, as healthier products are costlier than unhealthy products.

Since the determinants of health lie in many sectors, we need 'health in all policies'. To convert this from rhetoric to reality, we need to build capacity for health impact assessment and evaluate the potential and effects of policies and programmes in other sectors on human health and wellbeing. Health-impact assessment needs to be promoted on the lines of environmental-impact assessment. It needs to be multidisciplinary in its approach and assess both direct and indirect health impacts. The UN Sustainable Goals provide an actionable blueprint for multi-sectoral efforts to correct the distortions of development that pose threats to human health and wellbeing.

It is also necessary to bring people's voices prominently into such assessments. While it is often argued that 'health in all policies' will remain an aspirational slogan rather than an operational reality, if policy coherence is not mandated and monitored at the highest level of governance, alignment has to occur at multiple levels. The determinants of health must be moulded by the people who are most likely to be affected by their effects, not by unbridled market forces that are only attracted by financial profits.

We need to create powerful coalitions of people's representatives and civil society organizations which can advocate for, and monitor progress in, adoption and implementation of health friendly policies in all sectors.[28] Experiencing health as the product of several policies is the daily lived experience of the people. Nutrition-sensitive policies, for instance, which span across water, sanitation, food systems, education and gender equity, are influenced by people's legitimate expectations and powerfully articulated civil society voices. Operational alignment of services in these and related sectors is best gauged and glued at the community level.

A Scaffolding for Rebuilding
Public Health Services in India

Imrana Qadeer

Introduction

At a time when most things seem to be falling apart except for divisive forces, the hope for rebuilding one sector of welfare seems irrational. Yet, the desire to reform public health requires articulation as a part of the larger struggle for rebuilding democracy. To do this, we need to look back, dig out overlooked evidence and redraw lessons from history. Moreover, we need to understand the requirement for rebuilding public health in its integrated conception.

Classically, public health was defined as the 'science and art' of organized promotive, preventive, curative and rehabilitative health care by a collective effort of the people.[1] Global advances in organized medical care and technology, over time, influenced this vision and the Institute of Medicine's 1998 report, *The Future of Public Health*, defined public health as an organized community effort to address public interest in health by applying scientific and technical knowledge to prevent disease and promote health.[2] This emphasis undermined the social nature of public health and diluted the 'art' of public health practice—essentially democratic in nature. The shift towards a technocentric approach to health care later penetrated the WHO as well, which, while acknowledging developmental and welfare factors as crucial, played up medical determinants and the role of and access to technology in public health.[3]

This essay attempts to understand the complex nature of public health. Its underlying assumption is that public health is not achievable in isolation; one must adopt a perspective that encompasses an economic and social policy frame. India does not need to wait to acquire all the modern medical technologies to achieve comprehensive universal health care. It can draw from its positive and negative experiences to build missing links and construct a suitable scaffolding for public health in the country. This essay explores the principles of integrated planning in health care that were introduced by the architects of early planning in independent India but neglected later. It illustrates the innovative strategies that attempted to regain ground in this regard in the 1970s and early 1980s and how the growing influence of national and global structural adjustment policies and the post-1990s health sector reforms scuttled these efforts. These so-called reforms led to the privatization, commercialization and rising cost of medical care, transforming it into a commodity and a revenue-generating entity. In the process, the goal of basic health care for the majority got marginalized. The negative implications of these limited reforms have been highlighted by the COVID-19 pandemic. This essay draws its lessons from history and the current experience of the pandemic to re-evaluate future health care planning.

Complexity as the Essence of Public Health

Classical epidemiology—the basic science of public health— offered a comprehensive perspective for understanding causality of disease by pointing to a multiplicity of variables. It was, however, limited, as it had no way to measure the role of these interlinked variables. Statistical techniques came to its rescue by offering ways to prioritize and select variables and to measure the strength of relationships between various determinants of health and health status. In the process, however, these techniques very often distorted the problem itself to fit the tools of analysis.

Health sciences have struggled to find ways out of this block. Advances in statistics, chaos theory and operations research that deal with complexity have brought new insights in dealing with complex and dynamic nonlinear systems like public health. While chaos theory has underlined the importance of context and the initial conditions of a state of being (in health or disease), it has also underscored that in a complex, dynamic system, projections for the future have their limitations and are never perfect. An interesting insight it has offered is that dynamic systems can break or acquire new forms in their evolution and the transitions can be chaotic. Yet, vague patterns become perceptible which are the precursors of future trends. Hence, a minute change in initial conditions may lead to radically different shifts. Often, they can show us the way and offer choices if one is serious about the need for change. It has helped epidemiologists understand that though epidemiology primarily deals with a population-level subsystem, it is also influenced by molecular, social, political, environmental and market subsystems. In other words, epidemiology must see populations as complex social systems and not as a simple conglomerate of discrete individuals, as is often done in statistical analysis bereft of a social perspective for the study of human societies. Also, public health planning apart from the use of epidemiology requires medicine and biomedicine, social sciences, discipline of administration and organizational management, financing and policy studies.

Operations Research (OR) evolved in the acquisition of mathematical perfection of machines, moved into dealing with issues of post-war European reconstruction and then, market management where it offered methods of cost saving and increasing efficiency of complex systems. Here too, complexities of human systems forced researchers to move from mathematical precisions to probabilistic models that opened up options and choices as well as the debate on the pervious nature of boundaries of open systems. It enriched public health thinking by offering forecasting, a way to deal with uncertainties, unknowns and the inherently conflicting demands within public health systems. It ensured that systemic directions were monitored and ideological underpinnings boldly stated as against the acclaimed objectivity of scientific research.[4] It thus emerged as an alternative way of solving problems of complex systems. How much of these ideas were used in planning is what we explore below.

Early Years of Indian Planning

The exciting as well as promising knowledge of theory of complexity came to academic debates in public health mostly after 1970 and reverberates in many of its discussions. It is interesting therefore to look at the history of planning in India and discover that the Indian architects of planned development were not only aware of complexities (in a general sense) but also talked of integrated planning and use of OR to solve problems.

Mahalanobis, working closely with Nehru for the Planning Commission, envisioned his expertise in statistics as a new technology to increase the efficiency of human effort by using numbers and knowledge. He believed that planning must be based on a progressive and integrated economic policy, rather than reliance on a number of useful but unconnected projects.[5] Under Mahalanobis's guidance and Nehru's oversight, the second Plan (1956) used OR and optimization.

Mahalanobis opined, 'I have been using the phrase "operational research" in relation to planning in India. Our aim is to solve the problem of poverty, that is, to find a feasible method of bringing about a continuing economic development of the country. It would be necessary to use much scientific and technical knowledge and also to organize continuing research at various levels for this purpose. But research is not our primary objective; the aim is to solve our particular problem. When a practising physician gives medical treatment to a patient, he uses much scientific knowledge and may even do some research, but his chief aim is to cure the patient. His observations or experiments on the patient may add to medical knowledge but the treatment given is not primarily for purposes of research. The distinction is important . . . This is why I have used the phrase operational research in the present connection.'[6]

While underlining the importance of conceptual framework and models of complex systems in a practical exercise of problem solving, Mahalanobis was equally insistent that these have no permanent value. He used them 'as scaffolding to be dismantled as soon as their purpose has been served. There is, of course, much need of theoretical thinking and researches; but so far, we have been primarily concerned with practical issues, that is, with operational (as distinguished from theoretical) research'.[7]

As Mahalanobis envisioned it, the five-year plan would be flexible and always keep a long-term view wherein yearly plans would adjust for short-term experience. To achieve balanced growth, he said, the activities of the private sector must conform in a general way to the programme of production of the plan as a whole. A two-way information flow and data exchange between the Planning Commission and field projects would consolidate planned development. Though the focus was economy, conceptualization of OR had elements applicable to all sectors. These included visualizing the problem, identifying possible solutions and choosing the most appropriate one. Its application required monitoring and research to fill gaps in knowledge for acquiring balance and efficiency in the outcome of interventions. Also critical were rationalization of resource allocation for interventions and feedback into conceptualization as well as operations.

This intense effort at handling complex problems of integrated economic planning with distributive justice and people's consent was based on the broader perspective that Nehru offered—'of an ethical state endowed with the responsibility of modernizing a traditional country with the help of scientists and a scientific temper. A mixed economy where the state ought to play a great role in building the economic infrastructure'.[8] According to Pathak, Nehru dreamed of Big Industries (or 'Temples of New India'), science labs, institutes of technology and new universities for creating a resurgent human force that would be rational, secular and progressively nationalist. It would strengthen the pillars of liberal democracy with its periodic elections and help maintain a delicate balance of extreme political forces implicit in a country full of diversities. Nehru was very impressed by the Russian experience in handling the challenge of poverty and unemployment, which required mobilizing resources and providing welfare, especially education and health. Yet he was aware of the limits of the Russian experiment, which he wished to avoid, even at the cost of lower growth rates. Hence, his idea of India was based on democratic socialism, planning and industrialization, increase in food production through structural reforms and commitment to secular credentials. He imagined a welfare state with the consent and confidence of the people in a democratic socialist political economy of planning and decentralization.[9]

There are critics of the Nehru–Mahalanobis strategy of planning within and outside the country but there is no denying that India did acquire a growth rate of 4.1 per cent with remarkable structural shifts in agriculture and significant reduction in economic inequality over the Nehru years of 1951–1964.[10, 11] This was quite distinct from the post-1990s jobless growth with rising inequality.

There were of course significant limitations in implementation, since records tell us of insufficient land reforms and employment generation, food grain shortages, industrialization that barely induced growth impulses, and non-Plan years of the late 1960s in the Indian economy. The Sixth Five Year Plan in its review of social justice over the two decades—1960s and 1970s—showed that while the share of the rural poorest 30 per cent in consumer expenditure moved up from 13.1 per cent to 15.1 per cent, the urban poor did not gain even this much. The assets of the lowest 30 per cent rural population had in fact slid from 2.5 to 2.0 per cent. Only the lowest 10 per cent remained where they were.[12] This was the first and the last such review by the Planning Commission and the Seventh and the Eighth plans were already pushing for privatization—shifting from total coverage to targeting of the poor.

Conflicts of Faith in Technology and the Biases Inherent in Social Structure

As Nehru and Mahalanobis attempted to implement their plans for economic and social development, they held the strong belief that science and technology could break all social barriers despite their deepening understanding of poverty and politics. Within the broader Nehru–Mahalanobis perspective, rapid increase in health care and a national health service was visualized with priority to full coverage with basic care instead of high-quality care for a few. Thus, paid health assistants in charge of a group of villages would function under fully trained physicians, and facilities for medical training would be increased in urban areas.[13]

However, the interests of the ruling caste-class combined with its gender biases deeply entrenched in the political structure was not easy to overcome, and are reflected even now in economic and health policies such as the labour laws or the ASHA workers' constant struggle for recognition. The impatience of the ruling caste-class combine undermined planned development by resisting land reforms, expansion of public sector enterprises, creation of jobs, providing living wages, universalization of school education, building primary health-care infrastructure and a progressive perspective towards public health. Investments in the welfare sector as a whole declined, with investment in the health sector specifically getting reduced from 3.2 and 2.9 per cent of the GDP in the First and Second Plan to 2.1 and 1.9 per cent in the Fourth and the Fifth Plans (excluding family planning).[14] Till date, they have not touched the previous 3 per cent of the initial plans or the promise of the National Health Policy 2017.

The soft attitude of the committed elite towards biases inherent in social structure is also reflected in the earlier planning documents for health. The report of the Committee for Health and Development-1946 which was adopted post-Independence as the blueprint for health-care development, saw the observed 'apathy' of the people towards their own ill-health as the cause of 'continuance of the existing state of affairs through many generations'.[15] This understanding was superficial as they blamed people's tolerance for their conditions but did not identify the common roots of their tolerance—apathy and non-participation rooted in caste, class, religion and gender-based exploitation. Nehru and Mahalanobis considered these barriers surmountable. They saw the welfare objectives of the Second Plan not simply as an end in themselves but as part of a greater integrated project of overcoming the social constraints through economic growth, modernization and industrialization, and they believed they could carry this conviction through.

The Decades of the 1970s and 1980s

A series of substantive programmatic interventions to expand and strengthen health service infrastructure were made initially that we discuss below, but these could not survive in an overall socio-economic frame where equality, inclusive processes of development, individual rights and genuine participation became secondary to economic growth. The elite nature of growing markets and technologies marginalized these interventions that might have been the harbingers of a new India.

In 1978, India was a signatory to The Alma Ata Declaration of Health for All by 2000. This declaration attempted to usher in Comprehensive Primary Health Care (CPHC), health based on subsistence, welfare, acceptable and affordable technology, self-sufficiency and people's participation. Once again India's CPHC became a pale shadow of the political concept of CPHC. It was transformed into selective PHC after the World Bank exercised its heavy hand and WHO proposed that developing countries need to choose their targets selectively for problems for which technology is available and leave out issues of subsistence as they are long-term challenges. The focus was further narrowed to maternal and child health, and to reduce population numbers. Though defined as 'essential services', universal immunization, contraception and maternal and child health services were centre stage.[16] Though narrowed, these services were still considered the responsibility of the state.

However, in the 2000s in the name of Universal Health Coverage, a more nuanced strategy for releasing the state from its responsibilities was proposed. 'Coverage' was offered, not 'care'; with the partnership of the private sector to which resources could be transferred in the name of compensation for services (Chakravarthi 2019).[17] Granting autonomy to district hospitals meant that the referral links with the peripheral primary level services were broken. Their self-sustenance required entering the market, providing services that generated revenue and not services that were a national priority.

Rural Community Health Workers (RCHWs), trained volunteers who served as people's representatives to monitor health services and serve people, were introduced in 1977. Select literate villagers were trained to do basic health work. The idea was to train

100 CHWs per primary health centre per year, covering all the 5.8 lakh villages each with a CHW in two years. An equal number of traditional midwives were to be trained by the Lady Health Visitors to serve each village. This scheme was to run with the help of panchayats and people in selecting, monitoring and supporting the CHW. The scheme had potential, but its conceptualization and implementation did not account for the many problems that similar schemes faced earlier. The trainers were themselves inadequately trained in rural health-care management. Absence of strong district support and inadequate guidance made the CHWs subordinates of the health services rather than a voice of the community. Many turned into self-appointed private practitioners. Additionally, the social stratification led to biased selection, favouring the upper castes, who neglected the poor and the SC/ST communities. The neglect of basic social and organizational issues relegated the scheme to the margins and the opportunity to create a strong people-based participatory process in the delivery of grassroots services was thus lost.[18] Accredited Social Health Activists (ASHAs) replaced the CHW in the 2000s. These are women who look after reproductive, maternity and child health. The scheme suffers almost all the ills of the CHW scheme. The workers continue to demand formal integration into the health services and higher remuneration given the heavy workload and poor working conditions.[19]

The Reorientation of Medical Education (ROME) scheme was initiated in 1977. Its objective was to involve medical colleges by encouraging the adoption of Community Development Blocks across the country and participation in preventive, promotive and curative health care in PHCs.[20] The idea was to strengthen district services and make undergraduate education more sensitive to CPHC needs. The departmental involvement of faculty members was to extend this sensitization beyond Community Medicine departments. This very critical scheme failed to take off as CPHC itself never became a reality. The faculty could not be motivated and students found these postings unexciting due to lack of facilities and teachers. Though selected institutions continued to run useful community-based limited projects through their community medicine departments that encourage both students and faculty to explore challenges of CPHC and handling medical care in rural areas,[21] the experiment of actual participation in district health-care systems failed due to the apathy of medical college authorities, resistance and disinterest of faculty and health administration.

The Universal Immunization Programme of 1985 was the consolidation of immunization strategy following the control of smallpox. In 1992, it was assimilated into the Child Survival and Safe Motherhood Programme, and then in 2005 into the National Rural Health Mission. Despite these attempts at integration, the fourth round of the National Family Health Survey (2015–16) showed that only 37 per cent of children were fully immunized, 56 per cent partially and 7 per cent never immunized. There is a disproportionate concentration of immunized children in higher wealth quintiles, demonstrating a socioeconomic gradient in immunization.[22] It is evident that the deteriorating infrastructure for PHC and ICDS services are responsible for this deficit. Moreover, instead of first making the basic immunizations available, the strategy today is to push new and expensive vaccines, irrespective of both their value and questions raised by scholars.[23] Force and threats of denying school admissions to children are being used to push this technology thus transferring the onus on to parents rather than the health system, which must first demonstrate safety and effectiveness.

The laxity and distortions in these interventions show how health sector reforms in India actually serve the interests of business at the cost of the majority and how public health has become a victim and a vessel for market expansion.

The Dream of Rebuilding Public Health in India

The health sector reforms post-1990s were welcomed by a section of the upper castes and classes who already had their basic needs fulfilled and easy access to welfare services critical for CPHC. They took these for granted and demanded tertiary medical care. Thus, propelled by the pressure for reforms as well as for international standards, these initiatives distorted, fragmented and commercialized health services. These reforms did away with the integrative planning process and overlooked the importance of non-medical services for health.[24] Moreover, State investments in the health sector in India not only declined to the lowest in the world but were shifted over to the private sector through various mechanisms such as public–private partnerships, concessions offered to the private sector and the shift of personnel trained in the public sector. Apart from rollback in investments, it meant no accountability, responsibility or transparency required of the private partner, except the expectation to generate revenue and add to the GDP.[25, 26] Inviting foreign investment into drugs, the hi-tech medical equipment industry and tertiary care meant higher shares in these enterprises for the corporate sector, further distorting priorities as controls slipped into corporate hands. Agricultural profits were diversified through investments in setting up hospitals and medical colleges—transforming them into a business.

The unsuccessful programmes discussed earlier are the products of this dynamic of socio-political and economic processes. The ongoing COVID-19 pandemic has exposed the weaknesses of the health service system—where the public sector is unable to cope, and the private sector uses illness as an opportunity for more profits. There is no transparency about resource mobilization and management and little concern for people's participation based on rationality and awareness. The state's use of draconian laws, police for public health work, and neglect of even the health providers has not helped either.[27]

Despite the official claims over the past three decades that there is no alternative but health sector reforms, an alternative set of reforms today is an imperative. This, however, can only be achieved as part of a mode of development where issues of livelihoods, living wages, equality of opportunities and individual rights are central to economic planning, and compassion and conflict resolution guide policy. Rebuilding public health is possible only within a framework that helps rebuild lives, contributing not only monetary but social profit—the health of the people whose economic value is accepted though never estimated.

Public health requires a cadre of public health practitioners like the cadre for administrative services[28] who are well trained in the interdisciplinary approach to this discipline. Medical education must be reoriented so public health is taught as a science and art of organizing health care for a people by their collective praxis, inclusive of but not controlled by experts, bureaucrats or international advisers. Social sciences must be incorporated not as a mechanical routine (as is often done in medical colleges), but as a way to make students sensitive to the complexities of public health practice and administration. Exposure to history and politics of public health furthers such sensitization. To grow, this discipline must cross the boundaries of community medicine departments, draw in other clinical departments into their field areas and together, evolve ways of tackling health-care challenges in large populations. Reorienting education[29] and rebuilding services calls for realizing that technology devoid of a social basis for its application can become a monster that controls and destroys, not heals, as demonstrated by Illich who highlighted the data for the US on the negative effects of medical care—physical, social and cultural.[30] Nundy, Desiraju and Nagral's edited volume reflects the pervasive malpractice and its consequences in India.[31] Training of primary care providers for peripheral institutions, which has remained neglected for long, is equally critical.

In rebuilding public health, strengthening primary health-care infrastructure, its referral chain and components are critical. Therefore, forming appropriate community-based monitoring systems with genuine participation of different sections is essential. The private sector must either be compelled to conform to the conditions of partnerships or stand for itself. It must be made accountable for the responsibilities it accepts, and a level playing field promoted in its partnerships with the public sector. This requires that efficient regulatory mechanisms for both public and private sectors are built into the system. Traditional systems of medicine (AYUSH)—used by a large section of population—have to be given their place in health care, not as a substitute for absent allopathic practitioners but as alternative ways to health and healing as envisioned by eminent medical practitioners and planners as early as 1929 at the All-India Medical Conference at Lahore.[32] Inevitably, adequate investment is called for in the public sector, which has been denied its due till now. Lastly, health is a state subject and must remain so without any distortions.

We have these pieces of a shattered dream of health services lying around, of the post-Independence efforts, of CPHC and its elements, of a public system providing health for all, of collective community action for health and of bringing medical students closer to the reality of this country. Past experience provides us lessons. The problem with picking up those pieces is that they would not fit within the contemporary socio-political reality. How can people live with security, dignity and the freedom to exercise constitutional rights and practise democracy so that they can pick up the scattered pieces and reconstruct a lost dream with their very own creativity and imagination? This possibility is being explored in some rural field experiments using public health itself as a first step. For example, through district level community-based monitoring and planning in Maharashtra[33] and community-centred health care in underserved rural areas of Bilaspur.[34] The 'unfolding unknown' in the complexity that was health planning of the 1950s is no more so, since understandings from history of planning and health services development tell us that it is the structural constraints that deny a large section of citizens those very basic conditions and services that are fundamental to achieving health. Addressing the structural constraints is central to rebuilding public health.

Innovation in India's Health Sciences: Three Pathbreaking Examples

Darshan Shankar, Chethala N. Vishnuprasad,
Gurmeet Singh, Varnita Mathur and Madhumitha Krishnan

Introduction

It may perhaps surprise the reader and cause wonder as to why this essay begins with an exposition on 'tradition and modernity' followed by views on the 'plurality' of knowledge systems. We hope that as the reader engages with this essay, this surprise transforms into a critical engagement appreciation or critique of the standpoint of the authors.

It is historically and sociologically evident that generation, transmission and transfusion of knowledge across cultures has occurred, and deep knowledge systems and their applications in many domains ranging from mathematics to culinary arts and medicine have been transferred. It is the politics of knowledge, in particular historical periods, that mainstreams some and marginalizes others.[1] In the context of marginalization, sections of Indian intelligentsia, to quote a phrase used by Ashis Nandy, continue to nurture 'colonized minds'[2] that overlook the strengths within their own cultural and intellectual traditions. A typical example is regarding the very notion of modernity. Seeded during colonial rule, a big sociological myth has been perpetuated about the dichotomy between tradition and modernity.[3] These were projected by the colonizers as polar opposites in order to spread the false idea that India needed to import modernization from the West. In fact, tradition and modernity lie on a continuum. Much as the past, present and future lie on a continuum, the present being derived from the past and the future from the present, so also do the roots of modernity lie in tradition. Historically it is observed that the normal sociological process by which a culture modernizes is by building on its traditions. The modernization process of Europe in the fourteenth century is an example because it is well known that the Renaissance drew its inspiration from classical Greek tradition. This does not imply blind adherence to tradition. Adjustment of traditions to temporal changes happen. Modernization processes may include discarding, modifying and even innovating by making radical departures from traditional ways. But the reference for modernization is always the past.

A society's alienation from its roots is a distorted phenomenon and can happen in various political contexts. It can be observed in a new social formation like in the case of the United States, Australia, Canada and New Zealand wherein large sections of native leadership were killed and indigenous cultures marginalized. It can also happen to varying degrees due to an extended history of oppressive and aggressive foreign rule like colonialism, such as in several countries in Asia, Africa and South America, wherein the ruled populace was so culturally and intellectually dominated, weakened and brainwashed that it has continued to look down on its own traditions, despite their contemporary potential and relevance. Even within a society the cultural impulses of minorities (e.g., tribals) can also be inhibited and weakened when they are suppressed by an economically and politically dominant mainstream.

* * *

In the context of health sciences, which is the theme of this essay, it must be recognized that while modern Western biomedicine (allopathy) introduced during the colonial period, with the support of biology, chemistry, physics and engineering, has achieved in a very short time remarkable outcomes particularly in diagnostics and surgery, its projection as the only viable mainstream is a colonial idea. The idea that the indigenous health sciences like Ayurveda need to be discarded in a modern society because their principles, concepts and methods are different from Western medicine, is of political origin. All knowledge systems, both Western and Indian, have their strengths and limitations arising from their world views. The scientific knowledge system despite its strengths, is recognized to be reductionist in nature. This is because it is based on an atomic and cellular perspective of physical and biological reality. Today scientists at the frontiers of knowledge recognize that an understanding of biological changes at a cellular and molecular level can simply not be extrapolated at the level of tissues, organs and to the whole biological system because of the complex patterns of cross talk across cells within tissues, organs and the interconnectedness of the human biome. Its very method for study of nature in laboratories has limitations because no science laboratory (however sophisticated) can mimic the complexity of the physical or biological world. It can only create models that give an extremely reduced view of the world.

In classical Ayurveda, nature is observed directly by minds trained in sankhya (a profound method of observation), yoga (an experiential knowledge of interconnectedness), nyaya (logical system quite different from Aristotelian logic), not at the molecular level but in terms of the ever-changing macro changes in five states of nature which are aakash (empty space), vayu (gaseous), agni (heat, plasma), jal (liquid) and prithvi (solid). This Indian perspective has given rise to specific health science-related categories for observing systemic biological changes like tridosh vichar (systemic physiology), dravya guna Shastra (systemic pharmacology), dashvid-pariksha (ten biological and ecological parameters for holistic diagnosis), kaya chikitsa (algorithm-driven treatment principles that address variability) and several other subjects that are beyond the scope of this article.

In fact, the terms Ayurveda and biology both carry equivalent etymological meaning in two different languages, Sanskrit and Greek. Both the terms mean 'the study of *changes* in life processes'. Despite this common goal, the principles, concepts, methods of observation and techniques are very different. The difference is on account of the systemic perspective (panchmahabhut siddanth) of Ayurveda versus the molecular perspective in biology. Their relationship is that of whole and part which are evidently interrelated. The relationship is however not one to one because the whole is not equal to the part and vice versa. In the last two decades very interesting research combining Ayurveda and biology has been underway and has given rise to exciting outcomes.[4]

Naturally the knowledge constructed on different foundations cannot look the same in terms of concepts, principles, methods and products. However it is marvellous to note that *order, change* and *complexity* in nature is observed both in macro (systemic) and micro (molecular) expressions of nature evident in the construction of sophisticated systems of knowledge like Ayurveda and biology.

Universal values embodied in a knowledge system is an indication of its applicability across space and time but it is not only European sciences that possess the monopoly to lay claim to universality. There are several examples of universal knowledge transferred from Asian, African, South-American and European cultures that have significantly transformed theoretical, technological, natural resources and aesthetic domains in the borrowing culture.

The test of the competence of any knowledge system is not based on its epistemology (way of knowing) and ontology (the reality it uncovers), but on an assessment of whether its theory and practice and its understanding of nature and society, can consistently be applied to transform and solve real-life problems. Solutions and their mode of action are bound to be different across knowledge systems. To reject and ignore a solution because its logic is different from a particular dominant knowledge framework is sheer prejudice and ignorance of plurality. Every functional knowledge system possesses strengths and limitations and hence plural approaches can have unimagined benefits if they are combined in epistemologically informed ways that compensate for the limitations of singular approaches.

To delve further into the epistemological argument outlined above, it is necessary to enquire if Ayurveda, Yoga, Siddha (Tamil medical system), Sowa-Rigpa (Tibetan medicine), Unani and other non-mainstream Indian knowledge systems that operate in parallel to Western medicine in India really work. Outside the mainstream biomedical health system, the Ayurveda and Yoga knowledge systems have the largest and most rapidly growing health-care infrastructure in India. This essay will, therefore, purely on grounds of pragmatism, focus on Ayurveda.

A caveat however must be admitted at the outset. There is, undoubtedly, limited published recent research data on the effectiveness of Ayurveda. The reader may note that the quantum of research data is directly a function of investment in data collection. The absence of data is the result of negligible and pathetic clinical research investment by the government. It is not due to choice or inclination of Ayurveda practitioners. At the same time it is significant to note that despite limited published evidence about its effectiveness, Ayurveda's phenomenal growth post-Independence appears to be on account of public acceptance of its health services.

The growing consumer acceptance and apparent effectiveness of Ayurveda clinical services in India is observable from two data points. Firstly, Ayurveda industry (manufacturing and services) growth trends. Its current size is estimated in 2022 to be around 40 billion USD.[5] The second source of information is from the limited clinical research studies in the public domain. Published case studies exist that demonstrate that Ayurveda possesses the ability to manage complex health disorders of human, animal and plant systems. A striking example of Ayurveda's clinical performance in COVID times, was its ability to manage conditions attributed to microbial infections (black fungus) without the conventional strategy of antibiotics. A recent case study in an Ayurveda clinical establishment demonstrated its ability to treat pulmonary mycosis, a recurrent fungal infection, successfully.[6] This ability has also been observed in other infectious conditions ranging from fevers to diarrhoeas, gangrenous wounds, UTIs, Herpes zoster and amoebic dysentery. Clinical evidence also shows the 'antiviral' role of Ayurveda in viral infections like dengue and chikungunya. A number of cytotoxicity studies reported the immunomodulatory role of Ayurvedic herbs in improving platelet counts.[7] The detoxification procedures of Ayurveda (panchakarmas) are also observed to have remarkable outcomes on the metabolic and immune functions.[8]

Apart from health sciences like Ayurveda, Yoga, Siddha, Unani and Sow-Rigpa, with their sophisticated theoretical apparatus and codification in thousands of medical manuscripts, India also possesses a huge diversity of functioning oral traditions practised by ethnic communities residing in different ecosystems and providing primary health care at the grassroots. These are referred to in current sociological discourse as Local Health Traditions (LHTs). Guesstimates suggest a million grassroots carriers of oral traditions, (Source: LSPSS publication, Centre for Indian Knowledge Systems, Chennai, India) in the form of midwives, bone setters and herbal healers. The existence of LHTs in this century indicates faithful transmission of functional practices, passed down the centuries through an effective oral transmission system. From the large number of medicinal plants (around 6500 species) including recently introduced exotics and animal species (around 300), discovered by LHTs across the country, it is evident that this stream of multi-locale knowledge has been evolving (Source: Trans-Disciplinary University database on Medicinal plants www.tdu.edu.in). Multicentric surveys (ethno-medical) indicate that such local traditions have offered communities useful solutions for human, animal and crop health[9, 10] for generations.

From an Indian perspective, then, one of the creative strategies to revitalize health sciences and seed innovation in health care is to draw inspiration from the systemic knowledge perspectives underlying Ayurveda and LHTs and combine them with the molecular perspective of biomedicine.

In fact, this integrative strategy for the future of health care is a key recommendation of the latest National Health Policy (2017). The innovation potential of this multi-cultural or trans-disciplinary approach is tremendous. In this essay we shall outline three pathbreaking examples. The first we outline is a strategy for the mass personalization of food. The second idea is on the potential of developing a new theory of pathogenesis and the third is of an ecologically sound, green way of enhancing *last mile reach* of health security to millions of rural and, to a smaller extent, urban communities, by revitalizing community-rooted local health traditions.

Example 1: Innovation for Mass Personalization of Food

The most low-cost solution to unmet health needs is food, as it is the daily input consumed to sustain human life. Yet, food and drinking water are the most neglected basic human needs from the perspective of health sciences.

Since government policies on agriculture and food-processing systems and infrastructure are targeted to feed masses globally, these have focused exclusively on increasing yield to make food available at low costs.[11] This is, of course, important, but without balancing it with scientific endeavours to enhance nutritional values by wise selection of species, habitats (e.g., there are native species of rice rich in iron, similarly habitats with specific soil microbes, rainfall altitude play an important role in enhancing nutrition) and processes adopted for food production, it leads to a society plagued by chronic health diseases, resulting in a huge health cost burden over time. Processed food, which has criteria focused on the sensorial and stability, has more often than not led to decreased nutritional value. Diabetes, obesity, cancers and cardiac disorders are examples of health conditions partially impacted by food.

Furthermore, foods selected for agriculture and food processing have neglected thousands of ecosystem-specific foods of nutritional value.[12] This has led to loss in diversity at all levels—of cultivated plant species, varieties within species, loss of recipes to cook them and finally a loss of diversity of food on the plate.

The massive industrial scale of these agricultural and food systems has resulted in uniform diets and excessive consumption of a few foods, again leading to negative health outcomes over time. A comparison of the number of foods in the National Institute of Nutrition, ICMR (NIN) library with the traditional Ayurveda library of food ingredients gives a sense of this. The NIN database documents around 542 food entities, derived from 296 unique species. Of these, there are 328 plant-based food entities obtained from 169 unique species. However, an in-depth review of documented food traditions in Ayurveda[13] has revealed records of 763 food recipes with plant ingredients obtained from 512 species. This indicates a threefold higher phylogenetic diversity in our traditional food library. The undocumented foods consumed by ethnic communities across diverse ecosystems is perhaps several folds higher, with their properties yet to be studied.

With respect to food, advances in nutrigenomics show that genotype plays an important role in determining nutritional needs[14] and therefore food and nutrition needs to be personalized to genotypic variations. Significantly, there are recent studies that establish a correlation between genotypes and Ayurveda phenotypes.[15] Though the relationship of genotypes to foods suitable for a particular genotype is hardly understood, the Ayurveda system of phenotypes is clearly linked to specific compatible foods.[16]

Ayurveda has long advocated diversity and personalization in food. It achieves personalization at a low cost because the Ayurveda phenotypes are easy to assess and reliably connected to compatible foods. Ayurveda applies this relationship to advise on personalized diet in routine clinical practice. Mass personalization of food needs a logic (algorithm) that brings together knowledge from several disciplines (e.g., food and blood chemistry, microbiomics, epigenomics nutrigenomics and Ayurveda-biology) and variables (e.g., phenotypes, genomics). Bringing together this complexity in a logical fashion on a mass scale needs artificial intelligence and machine learning (AI and ML)[17] for integrating and generating individualized solutions.

This strategy can probably deliver high-quality nutrition and 'mass personalization of food' at scale. The trans-disciplinary approach will overcome shortcomings of food chemistry which influences but does not translate into nutritional values, because of the genetic, metabolic and physiological variability in consumers. Ayurveda phenotypes and food pharmacology fill the gap of food chemistry. Personalization of food, nutrition and, for that matter, medicine is indeed one of the major health challenges of the twenty-first century. India is in a unique position to design and execute this strategy.

Example 2: Integrative Theory of Pathogenesis

There is a possibility of developing a pathbreaking strategy for early detection of disease based on integration of Ayurveda theory of pathogenesis (*shad kriya kal*) and cell biology. This integrative view of disease progression will be an original Indian contribution to the world of medicine.

In modern biology achieving equilibrium of physiological functions (homeostasis) at a cellular level is important for the body's overall health and wellness. Each cell performs basic biological functions like growth, reproduction and death. These fundamental biological events in a cell are regulated through an intricate control system referred to as biochemical signalling. Therefore, a cell is defined as healthy when all the cellular infrastructure—plasma membrane, cytoplasm, cytoskeleton, golgi apparatus, endoplasmic reticulum, mitochondria, lysosomes, ribosomes and nucleus—work together to maintain a homeostasis in biochemical signalling. Similar cells work together as tissues and organs and form the functional parts of the body. Thus, besides the health of a single cell, homeostasis is important for maintaining systemic health through intercellular and intertissue communications. When this intricate regulatory circuit of a localized cell network is distorted, it starts to transduce unnatural and faulty signals, resulting in disruption of cellular homeostasis and the localized cells can be defined as 'diseased'.[18] These distortions in biochemical pathways can be caused either by intrinsic problems, like genetic variations and hormonal imbalances, or external factors like infections and allergies. Biochemical signalling from diseased cells will eventually alter the normal communications between tissue and organ systems and ultimately lead to a total disruption of body homeostasis and overall health. These alterations are expressed as various disease manifestations, from a simple fever to complex multifactorial diseases like diabetes and cancer.[19]

While molecular events at a cellular level are critical, the manifestation of a disease is more complex and is a cumulative effect of several independent molecular events happening in different cells and tissues. Most often, disease manifestation is more than the sum of these individual molecular events. While many of the molecular targets involved are being explored to develop management strategies for various diseases, the whole cycle, sequence and pattern of disease progression, at a systemic level, is poorly studied today. The current dominant paradigm of drug discovery is the identification of active molecules that are effective on a particular molecular target at cellular level. However this strategy is not successful, particularly in multifactorial diseases, as these individual molecular events do not necessarily reflect the overall disease progression at a systemic level.[20] This poses important questions in disease biology. How appropriately do individual molecular events reflect the complex pathophysiology of a disease? Is the targeted molecular drug approach adequate to address the complexities of multifactorial diseases like diabetes and cancer?

Some of the recent advancements in systems biology and network pharmacology indicate that even carefully selected single compounds (tested on lab models) may not exhibit desired clinical efficacy on human beings. This is because lab models do not capture possible pharmacological or biochemical networking that is happening in the disease progression and pathophysiology.[21] Large-scale genomics studies have also shown that single gene knock-outs exhibit very little or even no effect on the phenotypic or functional aspects of every genome. A network biology analysis reveals that deletion of individual nodes in a disease network will have little effect; a modulation of multiple proteins may be required for perturbing a particular phenotype. Andrew Hopkins (a drug discovery expert) observes that the reasons for decreased rate of new drug candidates being translated to effective therapies is more a problem of systemic logic than a technical or scientific one, because diseases are understood only at their molecular level.[22] It is imperative to have newer strategies of understanding diseases progression that work at both molecular and systemic levels.

Perhaps this is where the role of transdisciplinary approaches is important. Holistic health sciences like Ayurveda understand health and disease at a systemic and functional level. As per Ayurveda's theory of disease progression (shad kriya kal), there are six stages: Sanchaya (stage of accumulation), Prakopa (stage of aggravation), Prasara (stage of spreading), Sthanasamshraya (stage of localization), Vyakti (stage of manifestation) and Bheda (chronic stage). In the first stage, *Sanchayavastha,* there is an accumulation of *Doshas (infection/symptoms)* in their own specific regions. This stage arises due to an abnormal or improper lifestyle and diet and results in a general feeling of illness, such as stiffness, mild hyperthermia, feeling of heaviness in the body and lassitude. As the accumulated Doshas increase in their own specific regions, the next stage, *Prakopavastha*, is manifested where specific clinical symptoms based on the vata, pitta or kapha cause aggravation. This is also influenced by the phenotypic nature of the individual.

While Ayurveda understands these as systemic changes, it is hypothesize that the accumulation of toxins (doshas) is perhaps reflected at the cellular level as well. This would start altering the normal functioning of a healthy cell, as well as the tissue systems and they would start entering into the 'disease' phase. This hypothesis corresponds in the Ayurveda shad kriya kal theory to the second prakopavastha, when the cells become 'diseased' and start sending faulty signals (biochemical signals).

To continue with the hypothesis, in the third stage, Prasaravastha, the Doshas are further increased and begin to overflow and start moving to targeted regions, leading to their spread. In the prasaravastha, the faulty biochemical signal produced from 'diseased' cells and tissues systems is transmitted to the other parts of the body through various autocrine and paracrine signalling processes. As the body progresses to the fourth stage, *Sthanasamshraya,* the increased Doshas get accumulated in specific vulnerable regions, leading to early warning symptoms of disease before its full manifestation. At this stage, signs of fever, vomiting, etc., are observed. Following it is the fifth stage of *Vyaktavastha,* the stage where there is complete manifestation of the disease, causing inflammation, tumour, cyst, abscess, erysipelas. Further development of disease results in the last stage of infection, *Bhedavastha*, or the stage of complications where the disease attains chronicity and the treatment becomes complicated.

A physician trained in shad kriya can detect early stages of disease progression and thus serve and guide his patients effectively. As the famous saying goes—a stitch in time saves nine. The earlier the intervention is started, the better disease progression is prevented; the later the stage at which intervention is begun, the more difficult the treatment of the condition.

Can shad kriya kal and cellular biology work together to produce a new transdisciplinary understanding of pathogenesis? A one-on-one comparison of these systemic Ayurvedic concepts with one or more molecular events may be found to be untenable. However, these concepts can be logically correlated in an Ayurveda–biology framework. For example, the first stage of disease progression, accumulation of Dosha, is unique to Ayurveda and one will not find an equivalent concept or molecular event in modern biology. However, this can be mapped to pathophysiological events such as infection, autoimmune changes, defective digestion and metabolism etc. that accumulates one of the three Doshas (Vata, Pitha and Kapha).

There is research evidence from the new emerging field called ayur-genomics that suggests the viability of combining Ayurveda and biology to generate a new science. The experimental design of the studies that generated ayur-genomics is described below to communicate to the reader that cross-cultural studies to understand the uniqueness and variability in individuals has yielded innovative results. Originating from a pilot genetic study (HLA typing) on around seventy individuals, where it was demonstrated that specific genetic marker variations corresponded to the three Ayurveda phenotypes (prakrutis). Ayur-genomics has intrigued many researchers. A study published in *Nature* performed genome-wide analysis and reported genetic correlations to the prakriti constitution with unique gene marker associations. Likewise, a study of gene expression correlations with prakriti has identified biochemical pathway regulatory differences, providing a potential key for disease predictions on the basis of prakriti phenotypic traits. Researchers have also attempted psycho-neural correlations to prakriti types. An article compared the physiologic, physical and psychologic attributes in DNA (genes) originating with birth that are unique with a person throughout lifetime to inherent prakriti traits. The study reported genopsycho-somatotypic similarities, explaining that individual prakriti constitution originates with birth and remains constant. Similarly, big data analysis, biomarker discoveries, pharmacogenomic studies in relation to prakriti types have been recently validated with ayur-genomics in some reports. This shows the potential of the platform of cross-cultural research today referred to by a new discipline called 'Ayurveda-biology', coined by the eminent scientist Dr M.S. Valiathan.[23]

A similar creative cross-cultural research strategy is being proposed for an Ayurveda-biology research on pathogenesis wherein the goal is to identify biological markers underlying the six different stages of disease progression described in Ayurveda's shad kriya kal theory.

Example 3: A Fourth Tier of Health Care

The last three centuries have witnessed the evolution of the modern State and its systems of governance. The governance systems across countries provide for State-managed services for basic social needs like education, health and public transport. It is evident that the biomedical health services embodied in National Health Systems in India, have been by largely influenced by their colonial genesis. The destruction and erosion of *non-institutionalized* community-based and managed Local Health Traditions (LHTs) during the last two centuries appears to be caused by bias arising from the politics of knowledge, which, in the Indian context, generally manifests as low esteem and poor regard amongst policymakers for indigenous knowledge and its social management. Prior to colonial rule and the introduction of the British model of health-care delivery in India, the indigenous health services were being delivered both by the community in self-help mode (dadima ka batua) as well as through trained physicians (vaidyas, siddhas, hakims, amchis). The British health systems in the UK had by the eighteenth century begun to adopt a completely state-sponsored institutionally driven system of health care. The same system was seeded during colonial rule in India and subsequently adopted by the Indian government in 1947. It has weakened, though not altogether destroyed, the community-based, self-help health practices in millions of homes and thousands of communities. This partial destruction of community self-reliance in health care is perhaps a collateral damage caused by adopting an over-institutionalized system of governance for social functions like health care and education (which too was community managed before colonial rule).

However, in recent times the AYUSH policy of 2002, the National Rural Health Mission programme guidelines of 2005, the NHSRC (National Health Systems Research Centre, Government of India) study of 2010 on health-seeking behaviour in communities by Priya and Shweta and the National Health Policy, 2017, have all recognized the value of community based LHTs. Amongst the serious proponents for revitalization of LHTs in the country, is the University of Trans-Disciplinary Health Sciences and Technology (TDU), Bangalore. The University has built one of the country's most reliable database on medicinal plants and traditional knowledge, derived from classical texts of Indian systems of medicine and published reports on ethno-medical and botanical traditions. The table below depicts the incredibly large number of species (6581) used by classical and folk traditions across the country. Utilized for human, animal and crop health, these 6581 medicinal species are geographically distributed across all ecosystems, from the Himalayas to the coastal regions.

System of medicine	Ayurveda	Folk	Folk(V)	Homeopathy	Siddha	TCM*	Tibetan	Unani	Western
Ayurveda	1537	773	310	176	756	360	246	427	74
Folk	773	5215	283	161	771	672	186	330	80
Folk(V)	310	283	545	47	300	137	82	111	14
Homeopathy	176	161	47	489	145	128	69	136	102
Siddha	756	771	300	145	1147	289	209	334	59
TCM*	360	672	137	128	289	880	109	205	80
Tibetan	246	186	82	69	209	109	250	177	23
Unani	427	330	111	136	334	205	177	493	63
Western	74	80	14	102	59	80	23	63	190
Total 6581									

*TCM = Traditional Chinese Medicine

Number of medicinal plant species used in different systems of medicine

Source TDU, BOTMAST database 2012

The grey boxes highlight the total number of species used in different systems. Under each system column it is shown how many species of a particular system are common to other systems.

Local Health Traditions and their use of medicinal plants in fact address the emerging requirements of a new global paradigm called One Health. This is because medicinal plants in the community and in codified Ayurveda systems are not only used for human health. They are also used in agriculture (vriksh Ayurveda) and for animal health (pashu Ayurveda). The use of plants in agriculture was documented two decades ago (in 2000) by the Indian Council of Agricultural Research (ICAR). It launched the National Agriculture Technology Project (NATP), a nationwide project to collect, document and validate indigenous knowledge of plant uses for agriculture. The ICAR study showed that slightly more than 80 per cent of local, traditional plant-based agricultural practices were valid and about 6 per cent of the practices were partly valid. In summary, there was overwhelming evidence in favour of the validity of agricultural LHTs.

Similarly, it is seen that medicinal plants are also highly effective in animal health. Over the last ten years, TDU scientists in collaboration with the National Dairy Development Board (NDDB) have been training thousands of veterinarians in modern dairies from Punjab to Kerala in the use of medicinal plants for animal health, based on the knowledge in Pashu Ayurveda. This knowledge can make India a global leader in organic management of animal health for cows, goats, poultry and even domesticated animals like elephants, dogs and cats. The tables below indicate the enormous relevance of Pashu Ayurveda for replacing antibiotics commonly used for diseases of cows, which have detrimental effects on human health because of human consumption of animal foods.

Table 1: Feedback from various milk societies from National Dairy Development Board (NDDB), GoI, on the efficacy of Pashu Ayurveda (ethno-veterinary practices, EVPs) for nineteen clinical conditions in cattle.

No.	Clinical condition	Number of animals treated	% cure
1	Mastitis	38305	93.27
2	Indigestion	9212	90.68
3	Foot & Mouth Disease (FMD)	11669	93
4	Foot lesion	4388	92
5	Fever	51691	92.5
6	Diarrhoea	50015	96.72
7	Joint swelling	500	90
8	Bloat	1830	86.75
9	Udder edema	1982	95.49
10	Repeat breeding	4637	84.37
11	Deworming	5906	95.77
12	Wound	1335	83
13	Uterus prolapse	429	76
14	Retention of Placenta (ROP)	1128	74
15	Downer	999	76
16	Udder pox, warts	658	67.6
17	Teat obstruction	1134	75.5
18	Ectoparasites /Ticks	1401	93.57
19	Haemogalactia	1336	95.5

Table 2: Feedback from ABBOTT Pharma (A well-known American company), from February 2019 to August 2020

No.	Diseases		% cure
1	Mastitis	1165	93.34
2	Teat Obstruction	458	90.74
3	Pox/ Warts/ Cracks	342	82.24
4	Fever	67	100.00
5	FMD Mouth Lesions	159	100.00
6	FMD Foot Lesions/Wound	277	100.00
7	Bloat & Indigestion	186	93.95
8	Tick/ Ectoparasite	556	94.37
9	Worms	1402	97.23
10	Diarrhoea	823	95.37
11	Repeat Breeding	107	58
12	Metritis	4	100.00
13	Retention of Placenta (ROP)	47	73.08
14	Udder Edema	285	97.5
15	Blood in Milk	105	98.21
16	Lamness/ Bursitis		75.00

The classical literature of Ayurveda contains references (Charaka Samhita, Su.1.120) that point to the symbiotic relationship of Local Health Traditions and classical traditions of Ayurveda, Pashu-Ayurveda and Vriksh Ayurveda.

In reimagining health in the twenty-first century, it is possible and desirable to empower millions of citizens in managing primary health of humans, animals and crops by revitalizing LHTs. A 2020 initiative, supported by the office of the Principal Scientific

Advisor (PSA), Government of India, which lays the foundations of a citizens' portal on medicinal plants, is a step in this regard. The graphic below outlines the architecture of the portal.

This portal will have information on the occurrence of medicinal plants in every taluka, town, city and states of India. It will link species to their classical uses, LHT and, where available, modern pharmacological applications for human, animal and crop health. An interactive, multi-lingual portal, it will crowdsource experiences of local communities.

The portal will seed the development of an evolving fourth non-institutional tier of the National Health System to democratize and decentralize health care, empowering millions of citizens.

Citizens' Portal on Medicinal Plants and One Health

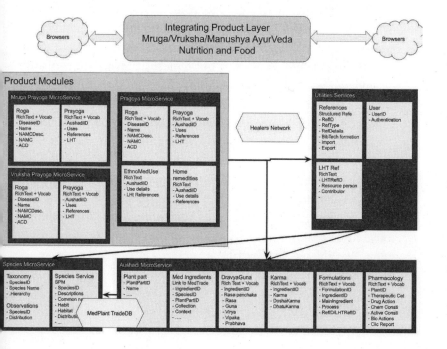

Concluding Remarks: An Action Agenda

This essay discusses three areas of innovations based on combining indigenous and Western sciences. The framework of Ayurveda-biology, however, has the potential to do more: for example, improve the classification of diseases, which today is not sufficiently sensitive to variability. It can enhance the quality of evidence generated by a reductive experimental and clinical pharmacology framework that is insufficient to understand complexity and variability in the human biome. It can also spur the evolution of holistic pharmacy models for drug discovery that use multiple molecule formulations and recognize the multi-factorial and syndromic nature of health.

This essay suggests that Ayurveda-biology has the potential to be at the core of 'integrative health science'. It can shape the new integrative health science of the future.

A new integrative science will expand the frontier of knowledge in health sciences by surmounting the limitations of Ayurveda's systemic understanding of biological change, due to its lack of tools to gain insight into changes at the molecular level, and similarly expanding the horizons of molecular biology which, given the complexity and interconnectedness of the human biome, cannot extrapolate cellular changes to larger biological systems in the body.

It must be pointed out that reimagining health sciences will need a new scheme of medical education that breaks the silos of medical knowledge systems. This is a complex task but essential to create a new cadre of health professionals with capacity to recognize strengths and limitations of different systems and promote integrative health practices when feasible, support innovative public health strategies and health research that bridges systemic and molecular biology of change.

Dreaming Health for All: Learnings from Civil Society Initiatives

Syeda Hameed

Introduction

As a member of the Planning Commission (2004 to 2014), my biggest challenge was to find solutions for the crucial sector with which I was entrusted, namely, health. Despite the thousands of crores spent on health over several five-year plans, the fact remains that the vast majority of our people continue to suffer; recurring illnesses take away whatever meagre little they own. If they don't die from disease, they die from the anxiety and penury that it causes.

Would the National Rural Health Mission, a flagship government scheme to deliver adequate and affordable health care to rural India, launched in April 2005, prove to be the panacea for millions of India's rural poor? Would a new Urban Health Mission rescue the urban poor from the trap of ill-health in which they are caught in the ever-growing slums of our cities?

I have always held one belief close to my heart. It is expressed best in this couplet:

Safar hai shart musafir nawaz bauhtere
Hazaar ha shajar-e-sayadaar raah mein hain

The condition is to keep travelling, there are many who are
hospitable
Thousands of shady trees line the journey

And this, indeed, is what I found. There were glimmers of hope in
hopelessness. Has anyone heard of Ganiyari, Gadchiroli, Ralegan
Siddhi, Akha, Sittilingi, Phek or Ehsaas in the metro cities where
policies are made and formulated as government schemes? Yet, was
health reaching these hinterlands where no government scheme
could reach?

What these people-centred health service initiatives of
physicians showed me was the possibility of what could be done
if we only galvanized our doctors' commitment and motivation.
They will then make it possible to create an ecosystem—of
medical education that inspires, and work environment that
facilitates such practice—that generates many doctors like
themselves. Would it be possible to provide motivated doctors in
the public system to innovate and practise as appropriate to the
diverse local contexts? Could they become the role models for
many more such civil society initiatives that receive government
support and facilitation? Even more importantly, can their work
provide pointers to envisage a different, more cost-effective
and people-oriented health-care system? Can that be the dream
fulfillment for a more effective, equitable and democratic health-
care system?

Whenever I despair and feel that I have reached a dead end,
something happens to lift my drooping spirit. So here is my journey,
over ten years of wandering.

Ralegan Siddhi: Pune, Maharashtra

October 2006

Eighty-five kilometres from Pune, in Ahmednagar district, is the village Ralegan Siddhi, best known for being the home of Anna Hazare. I drove there with a few friends in the early morning of 11 January 2005. I was working with my colleagues on the mid-term appraisal of the Tenth Five-Year Plan. The National Rural Health Mission had just been announced. The extensive consultations that I had held in preparation of the mid-term appraisal had revealed the work being done with community-based women volunteers. Trained and equipped by organizations such as Agragamee in Rayagada district of Odisha, Foundation for Research in Community Health (FRCH) in Parinche, Maharashtra, and Rani and Abhay Bang at Society for Education, Action and Research in Community Health (SEARCH) in Gadchiroli, these women were from the villages; they knew the people and were accountable to them. They were taught prevention and simple cures. I wanted to see how the model worked, whether it could be replicated all over the country and what this exposure did to the practitioners themselves.

The experiment had begun at Parinche village in the Purandar Taluka near Pune. Dr Antia, a physician and plastic surgeon, established FRCH at Mandwa near Mumbai to tackle the problem of health through a different kind of intervention. The idea revolved around treating illness not by increasing the number of doctors and nurses but by empowering village women to administer basic health care. Women volunteers were invited from the villages to work as Tais, Sahyoginis or community health workers. Though the idea faced initial resistance and shyness on the part of the women and cynicism by the men, it slowly took root.

To come back to Ralegan Siddhi, the training site was a short distance from the FRCH office and the village, in a wooded area.

When we reached, forty women were seated in a circle under a huge peepal tree. The sight exuded its own energy. A majority of them were young trainees from nearby villages. Their trainers were women known as Tais, who came from Parinche village, having been trained by FRCH. The women were to receive training in basic procedures such as taking blood pressure, drawing blood samples for haemoglobin testing, doing pregnancy tests, dressing wounds and administering simple medicines. They were also to be taught Ayurvedic, Unani and home remedies. Most of the teachers had ten years' experience. When we reached, we found them engaged in an Ayurvedic demonstration, boiling herbs such as lemongrass and spices such as cinnamon for upper respiratory problems.

The chabutra (a platform for community meetings) where the session was being conducted was near a mandir, a temple, which also served as an impromptu crèche. The voices of small children playing on the platform formed the backdrop of the training. At the end of their instruction, the women would receive certificates from the National Institute of Open Schooling in Delhi (NIOS).

As the women spoke, it became evident how the training had transformed simple village housewives into powerful members of the community. Today they were a force; their new avatar commanded the respect and deference of their men. Their voices tell their story best.

Nirmala Jagtap (Parinche village): 'I have studied till class IV. I have had ten years' experience, first as a Sahyogini, then as a Tai. First, I didn't like this work but then I realized that my knowledge about illnesses was helpful for my people because in my village there are no doctors. I used to approach people, now people approach me. I like my work. Even if the organization withdraws, I will continue.'

Pushpa Jadhav (Parinche village): 'We work to prevent diseases. We propagate use of clean water. We are trained in Arogya. We deal with microcredit. We advocate a clean environment. We wanted to build toilets because of the great need, so we went to our MLA and eighteen toilets were built.'

Kaval (Ramvadi village): 'I have studied till class IV. My village is isolated and there is no connecting road. Once, I examined a woman who had returned after her delivery and found her in terrible pain. I realized that part of the placenta had been left in the uterus. Her condition was dangerous. I contacted the doctor and asked him to come here and examine the woman or pay for the cost of transporting her from our village to his clinic. The doctor was initially very angry and asked for my credentials. I informed him that I was a certified Tai. He then apologized and came to Ramvadi and verified my diagnosis. The woman's life was saved. I was much appreciated by her family and many others.'

The trees around had notices pinned that gave important facts about the Right to Information Act. Forms, penalties and requirements hung on the tree trunks were emblems of the Ralegan Siddhi paradigm. Written in Marathi for the benefit of the women, they hung there, the simplest and most effective tools of empowerment.

For me, the crux of the experience was the inexorable truth that if women are empowered with knowledge about basic health care and hygiene and educated about Right to Information, they act as agents of change, who can achieve, much faster, the targets of our plans and of the Millennium Development Goals. The programme also worked as a tool for enhancement of their self-image; they became objects of respect in the village—their words were heeded by other women, the men and panchayats. Some of them told me how boys and men in their households had begun to help in the housework.

This is a case of social transformation that needs to be replicated on a much wider scale so that there are thousands of Ralegan Siddhis and hundreds of thousands of Tais spread through the length and breadth of the entire country. Tais are daughters of the village who have a personal stake in public health—no better way of ensuring the health and wellbeing of the poorest and humblest of our people.

Gadchiroli: Maharashtra

September 2006

Abhay and Rani Bang started SEARCH—Society for Education, Action and Research in Community Health in 1986 in the predominantly tribal district of Gadchiroli, Vidarbha. The idea was simple—Aarogya Samaj, a society where people's health is in their own hands. Brought up on Gandhian philosophy learnt in their early days at Sevagram, and armed with an MBBS and a master's in public health from Johns Hopkins University, this doctor couple began a battle to save thousands of neonates who die even before they get a chance to live. Shodhgram, the SEARCH campus ensconced in the verdant greens of Gadchiroli, 17 km from the district headquarters, was where the work began.

Shodhgram began from a small *tendu patta godown* in Gadchiroli town. Initial health surveys in hundred villages, especially among rural women, threw up alarming findings. The state of health and sanitation was abysmal. Prevalence of anaemia and malnutrition was high. Less than 5 per cent of deliveries took place in institutions and 56 per cent of the neonates delivered at home suffered from some morbidity. Just 2 per cent of them received medical treatment. Filariasis and malaria were rampant. The surveys documented high levels of reproductive health problems. Fifteen per cent of the population were carriers of sickle cell disease. Alcoholism and tobacco addiction was widespread. To reduce neonatal mortality, the Bangs began their intervention in thirty-nine villages. These villages were primarily non-tribal, chosen because the couple wanted to develop an intervention which would be applicable to all parts of the country, not just to the tribal areas.

In Bodhali, we met Anjana Uikey, a Village Health Worker (VHW) trained by SEARCH. Inside a small room, barely six feet by eight feet, covered with posters on child and maternal health, thirty-year-old Anjana recounted her triumphs and trials in her decade-long journey with SEARCH. She told us how she maintained a record of every woman in the village. 'Whenever a bride comes into our village, I make a note of it. Every two months, I check on all married women to find out whether they are pregnant. If they are, I register them and give them calcium, iron and folic acid tablets. I send them for antenatal check-ups, ensure that they take tetanus shots and advise them on the various aspects of pregnancy.' In case of an emergency, Anjana refers the patient to the Primary Health Unit in the village. This health unit has a doctor and, luckily for the women, also a lady doctor between 11 a.m. and 2 p.m. 'I try and do whatever I can,' said Anjana, pointing to a stack of neatly labelled bottles on a small shelf. Paracetamol, Salbutamol, Aspirin, Soda Mint—were all there. Health workers charged 10 paise per tablet and every transaction they made was meticulously recorded in a register.

In Bodhali, as in all the other villages in the area, most deliveries took place at home. So, when a woman went into labour, the health worker accompanied the Traditional Birth Attendant (TBA) to her house. These TBAs had also been trained by SEARCH and carried their own kits. Anjana told us that she assumed charge as soon as the baby was born. She washed, cleaned and checked the respiration of the baby, and also ensured that the mother started breastfeeding within half an hour of birth. Birth asphyxia, pneumonia and sepsis are universally acknowledged as leading causes of newborn deaths. Anjana proudly told us that she had handled nine cases of asphyxia, of which she had saved seven. With a doll, she demonstrated how she used a Mucous Extractor and Ambu bag to save asphyxiated babies. It was all done with pride and care. Strapping a watch on her wrist, she explained that timing was critical. 'I pump the Ambu bag forty times per minute for up to fifteen minutes. By then, if the child does not revive, I declare it a stillbirth.'

Anjana told us about the importance of family support in carrying out this work. Besides being a community worker, she had studied till class seven and worked as an agricultural labourer. As I saw Anjana confidently prepare her kit to do her rounds, I realized that the SEARCH experiment has done much more than saving the lives of babies. It has forever changed the lives of their mothers. Anjana told us that as per tradition, pregnant women were allowed to eat very little. 'It was believed that if the mother ate her fill, childbirth would be difficult and the baby would be born with a big head.' So, no food, no iron and folic acid capsules. Even after delivery, the woman was not allowed to eat eggs or vegetables for two months. 'When my elder daughter and son were born, my mother-in-law hardly let me eat anything. Then I joined SEARCH and realized how important nutrition was. When my third child was born, I put my foot down. Not only did I eat well, I resumed work within a week of delivery. This is what most women in the village do now.'

Seeing the bright faces of these children, we understood the importance of allowing health workers to use emergency lifesaving measures. The small team of saree-clad village women had vastly reduced neonatal mortality in their villages. These ordinary women had done the extraordinary. They were mostly in their thirties and forties, some a little younger, some older. Most had studied up to grade seven or a little more. They worked in the fields, cooked, cleaned and through sheer dedication, hard work, training and common sense, saved lives. They had brought about a slow and silent revolution in the most backward district of Maharashtra.

The kids who were playing near us would have been dead but for the Gentamicin injections given by the semi-literate village health workers. Their families would be bereft if the VHWs had not pumped life into them with their Ambu bags. Most women would have had to undergo multiple pregnancies while coping with the trauma of delivering dead babies. Given the frequent absenteeism of doctors, it is only these health workers who can help the children tread the thin line between life and death. They alone can reduce neonatal mortality because even if there is a doctor at the PHC, the child would never survive the journey from the village to the health centre. Both birth asphyxia and sepsis require immediate treatment. In Bodhali, we saw how this treatment can be effectively carried out on the spot by trained though semi-literate village health workers.

As we spoke to the women, they told us how they had saved babies who weighed just 800 gram; how the local PHCs and doctors now referred cases of sepsis and pneumonia to them; how the villagers only trusted the VHWs when it came to taking care of their babies. Manisha from Pardi village proudly informed us that when the village doctor's own child got sepsis, he trusted her to treat him. The women told us that even the 'jhola doctors' in their villages were happy to have them around because no one wants to touch a sick newborn baby.

The women told us about some traditional practices they had managed to change. One after another came the horror stories. Traditionally, till the umbilical cord fell, women were not allowed to step out of the delivery room. The placenta was placed in a pit inside the room and women had to clean themselves and answer nature's call in that very pit. This led to widespread infections, especially sepsis. Immediately after birth, the practice was to clean the baby with rice husk. The result was severe skin inflammation. Then the child was bathed with cold water to make her cry. No clothes were put on her for almost a month. We also learnt that for three days after birth, the child was only fed *gur paani*, jaggery water, not breast milk. The people feared that the mother's first milk was poisoned. The gur paani, however, led to diarrhoea. The VHWs admitted that most of their children had been born this way. Many had just died quietly. 'Now, we ensure that the child is cleaned, wrapped in warm clothes and breastfed within thirty minutes. The mother and family are instructed to clean and air dry their hands before touching the child,' said Chandrakala Kharvade from Dhonde Shiveni.

Abhay Bang explained the reasons behind the women's success where many experiments have failed. 'They are a part of the community. People have seen them save lives. They know that should any emergency arise, these women will be there with them. They won't be absent like the doctors and nurses in PHCs.' This trust was the key. It made it easier to give up ancient practices. The selection of the worker was crucial. For this, SEARCH followed a carefully conceived procedure. First, they laid out the minimum eligibility criteria and announced it in villages. When the applications came, they spoke to the families of the candidates, given the importance of family support. Thereafter, they consulted panchayats and village elders and shortlisted two to three candidates. These candidates were invited to the SEARCH campus. Through games, interactive sessions and plays, the potential of the candidates, their self-confidence and ability to respond under stress was gauged. Finally, the candidates were selected. Then began the process of training. Four to five days of workshops were followed by two months of field trials under supervision to gain practical experience. Six to seven such training sessions and the women were ready. Dr Bang informed us that of the 15,000 injections given by the workers, there has not been a single complication.

We left Gadchiroli with a feeling of cautious joy and hope.

Ganiyari: Bilaspur, Chhattisgarh

November 2006

I found further hope for health care in the form of a rural mission, Jan Swasthya Sahyog (JSS), running in a village called Ganyari, located in Achanakmaar National Park, 60 km from Bilaspur. At the turn of the century, in 1999, four men, doctors in their thirties, who had trained at CMC Vellore and All India Institute of Medical Sciences Delhi, felt an inner urge to give their skills and expertise to the poorest of the poor. Chucking up big pay packets and city lights, they moved to this forlorn tribal region. In this endeavour, they were advised by a former teacher, Dr B.R. Chatterjee, who had held a full professorship in Johns Hopkins USA, but had given up everything to settle in Purulia and shuttle back and forth to Chhattisgarh to remain in touch with his students. Another mentor was Dr Sathyamala, an epidemiologist who had studied at the London School of Tropical Medicine.

It was November 2006. Driving from Bilaspur to Ganiyari, set deep in the forest and remote, was like going back in time. With the Planning Commission team, I first went to the villages to look at JSS's Outreach Programme. The weekly clinics, run in several forest fringe areas, were attended by people from over 150 villages. Most of the people here were Adivasis; the majority were Gonds, and others were Baigas, Majhis, Oraons and Kols. Only a few villages were connected by all-weather roads. Most villages were inaccessible during the monsoons. So Ganiyari doctors needed to walk a few kilometres to reach their patients. It was an ordeal to travel by jeep to the village of Katani, where a crèche was running as part of the Phoolwari experiment. The other village we visited was Banhani, where we met Baiga and Gond women. Here, they had trained neo-literate and even illiterate women as health workers. In Banhani, women of all ages had come for training. Dressed in traditional attire and ornaments, they proudly showed us their small suitcases which were neatly stacked with medicines, breath counters for pneumonia detection, slides to take samples for malaria, dressing for wounds and pregnancy kits.

It was getting dark when we reached the abandoned irrigation building which had been leased for thirty years from the state government to run the referral centre, the outpatient clinic and the hospital ward. We could see how carefully the place had been restored. The natural ambience had been kept intact; inexpensive materials had been used. There were clean wooden benches, neatly numbered, lining the waiting area. The place smelt not of disinfectant but of fresh leaves. A sense of efficient orderliness was everywhere. In the referral area people were beginning to queue up. I learnt that they would spend the night there to get their turn early in the morning. I thought about the empty thirty-bed government hospital in the district headquarters, Kota, which we had visited enroute.

The OPD was packed with people even at this time of night. Some young women doctors were struggling with the case of an old woman who had been infected after a village quack had administered her an injection. The poison had spread. Doctors, unmindful of their personal fatigue and lateness of the hour, were attending to the woman and the distraught family. There was a seamless identification with people's suffering; just because they had darker skins and different features did not make their pain any less than that of patients at elite metro hospitals. For me, this was the most precious takeaway.

In the twenty-bed ward, the same sense of order prevailed: a woman with hysterectomy, a severe TB patient, a child with scalp surgery. I became aware of a young woman standing at the door. 'Sukhna Murmu. She is HIV-positive. Her husband died of AIDS. She dares not tell anyone. There is no ART (Anti-Retroviral Therapy) for her but we are trying.' The woman smiled at us and her wasted face lit up. Outside, an old hospital van was waiting to take the old woman to a private hospital for intensive care. 'This is Geeta'. The doctor pointed to a young girl. 'TB patient, but she has refused treatment. Her two older brothers died during DOTS.' Geeta was just five feet tall and weighed no more than 30 kg.

Through the course of the day and various presentations, it became evident to us that the low-cost technologies the doctors had developed could be used for a whole host of public health problems and detection of diseases. One by one these technologies were displayed. The Ganiyari method for early detection of UTIs cost less than Rs 2 per test, anaemia Re 1, diabetes Rs 2, pregnancy Rs 3. Most of these tests could be done by trained village women. I saw low-cost delivery kits, with everything needed for the mother and child—gloves, large plastic sheets, soap, disinfectant, blade, gauze, sterilized threads, cotton cloth to wrap the baby, thick sanitary pads for women to use in the first twenty-four hours. All this for Rs 40. There was a cheap and effective water purifier system; a person cycled for half an hour to draw several buckets of purified water. There was low-cost nutritional formula for severely undernourished children, much cheaper than that available in the market or in the public health system. They had perfected cheap technology to detect sickle cell anaemia and falciparum malaria. The list was long, the impact far-reaching.

For me, Ganiyari was a microcosm of rural India. 'It is in the vast expanse of rural India, where a majority of Indians still live, that the battle against disease will be won or lost.' How many times had I read these words? In Ganiyari, they acquired a meaning which had been eluding me all this time.

What lessons did I learn from Ganiyari? I learned about dedicated professionals who work directly with people to understand what ails them and what needs to be done both for prevention and treatment. These professionals had developed low-cost technologies which were effective. They used patients as partners in effecting their own cure, not as 'beneficiaries' who were a burden. They had placed faith in illiterate village women's ability to deliver health services and their belief had been vindicated. They used school buses and children as couriers to drop and pick up malaria slides to expedite the treatment. The sum total of all these interventions was that the poorest of tribals were for the first time getting decent health care.

The biggest problem that I have encountered in my field experiences is the unavailability of human resources in health. The one voice heard most often in villages is 'No doctor, no ANM (Auxiliary Nurse Midwife)'. The answer lies in recruiting from the community what the community can yield. The very act requires courage and faith. Can public institutions be made over from bureaucratically run institutions to people-friendly, service-oriented ones? The Ganiyari team reposed faith in the village women and reaped rich dividends.

Akha Ship of Hope: Dibrugarh, Assam

August 2007

Akha was a small ship, 22 m long and 4 m wide. It had a beautiful deck on which we rode. It also had an OPD, cabins for medical staff, a small kitchen, toilets, crew quarters and a general store. Sitting on the deck, watching the magnificent Brahmaputra River, we thought of the reach and grasp of the National Rural Health Mission that we had witnessed over the last two years.

'Have you ever thought about the chars (islands) in Assam?' Sanjoy Hazarika, the founder of Centre for North Eastern Studies (C-NES) had asked us in Delhi. 'Here, thousands of people live in adverse conditions, cut off from the mainland by a fast and furious river. The challenge is to give them access to basic health. How will they get sub-centres, leave alone Primary Health Centres? They don't even have drinking water.'

Our hour-long journey across the deceptively calm river was taking us to Dodhia sapori, a river island of Brahmaputra. On the river, we heard the rest of the Akha's story. In 2004, when the concept of a boat health centre was showcased by C-NES, it won an award at the World Bank's India Development Marketplace Awards. With the award money, the construction of the boat started. Carpenters from Dhola, Tinsukia worked tirelessly under the supervision of the engineer, Kamal Prasad Gurung. In June 2005, the ship that would bring hope to the lives of the thousands of forgotten char dwellers was completed. Since then, the Akha has made regular trips to these small riverine islands, organizing medical camps, immunizing little children and providing basic medicines.

Plodding through the khaironi grass, we reached the building where the health camp was being run. This multipurpose facility on stilts served as a school, an Anganwadi, and a health sub-centre. It consisted of one large room fronted by a verandah. When we reached, a few patients were waiting outside. Two hours later, the place was filled with people. Mishing (also called Miri) women, clad in bright shawls and sarongs that they had pulled up to mid-thigh, walked through the waist-length khaironi grass, babies strapped to their backs. They stopped to wash their feet at a hand pump. The doctors sat on the school benches, consulting patients across the desks. Nurses examined women patients in a corner and referred them to the doctors in the room. Medical supplies, neatly arranged on one side of the room, were dispensed by a pharmacist. The place was buzzing with life; health care had been carefully extended to the most deprived.

The C-NES, working in partnership with the government of Assam, the NRHM and UNICEF, has taken health care to the forgotten people on the riverine islands of the Dibrugarh, Dhemaji and Tinsukia districts of Upper Assam. Health care has thus reached 10,000 people, including many children who would otherwise have never been immunized.

Individual genius, which experiments and triumphs over adversities, is rarely used as a model for upscaling and replication. The government has the resources and the mandate to create a thousand 'Ships of Hope', which could bring health to people who are at the receiving end of a volatile and moody river. What it needs is the humility and willingness to learn from those who have successfully experimented.

Phek, Nagaland

2007

The idea of communitization was integrated into district planning by the visionary chief secretary of Nagaland, A.M. Gokhale, a first in Phek district. We saw it in operation in village Mopungchuket where the sub-centre is located. With 6000 people, most families have retired army men. It was one of the neatest and most aesthetic health centres we had seen in India, a tiny two-room wooden structure on the hillside. In one room were two neatly made beds, one of which was occupied by an elderly woman. Cheerful curtains hung at the windows, and flowers were laid on the stool next to the beds. Clean chairs lined the waiting area along with a few bowls of flowers. In the examination room sat a nurse who showed us her well-organized registers. Particulars of every patient who visited the centre had been recorded: name, age, ailment, treatment suggested and medicine given, all put down in a clear hand. Most of the patients, we noticed, were eighty-five years of age or more. 'What medicines do you give?' we asked the ANM. 'We try to provide the basics. The villagers all chip in with money to ensure that the centre is always well stocked and that no one in need is denied help,' she explained. I thought of the unhygienic (often closed) one-room sub-centres I had seen in states like Maharashtra, Uttar Pradesh, Rajasthan, Madhya Pradesh and Odisha. Those centres would never have been in such a decrepit state had the local community played a more proactive role in making them work.

Sitting in Delhi and making uniform policies for the country, it is hard to comprehend this health miracle at Phek. It is only a journey to the hinterlands that gives us the wisdom to recognize the discrepancies with reality and loopholes in our planning, as well as the many possibilities that exist on the ground.

Sittlingi: Tamil Nadu

August 2010

The Tribal Health Initiative (THI) Centre at Sittilingi is housed in a few single-storey, well-designed bamboo, cane and mud buildings spread across a quiet and clean campus. In 1993, Regi George, an anaesthesiologist, and Lalitha Regi, a gynaecologist, visited this area. He was a Kerala Christian, she from a Hindu family of Kochi. They wanted to work in rural India and were travelling to find the right spot. What they saw in Sittilingi shocked them. Mostly a tribal area, Sittilingi was so remote that, during the monsoons, it was completely cut off. People had no access to health care. Their traditional practices, like keeping the woman and child out in the cold at the back of the house for a week after childbirth, resulted in high maternal and child mortality. As the child survival rate was low, family size was normally six or seven. The doctor-couple had found the place they were looking for. 'We encroached on some land and built a mud-and-thatch hut with the help of the tribals. For three years, we ran a hospital from there. We managed to provide some care but, by and large, the problems persisted as the impact of our work did not change the retrograde practices being followed,' explained fifty-year-old Lalitha, clad in a simple salwar kameez. So, they started mapping the households in the village.

In 1995, they asked the villagers to select elderly women who could be trained to provide health care at the local level. Twenty-five women were selected from twenty-one hamlets. Every two weeks, these women would visit the centre for two days to learn the basics of health, hygiene and disease management, and to update the data about births and deaths in their villages. These women became the health-care providers and change agents in their tribal hamlets. At the time of our visit, there were twenty-three health auxiliaries in the forty to seventy age-group who received Rs 700 per month as a stipend and worked for two-three hours daily. Most were not literate but after training they were able to explain the basics of health and hygiene. As they were elderly, and from the community, people listened to them. We met some of these women, wrapped in cotton saris, standing outside the health centre. Among them was a younger woman, Rajamma. She had joined the doctor-couple when they first came to Sittilingi. 'I was sixteen years old and had dropped out of class eight,' Rajamma recalled.

'I started as a daily wager when the centre was being built but went on to learn nursing and assisting in deliveries. Now, I work as a nurse. I have even assisted in minor surgeries,' she said, her voice confident despite her uncertain smile. Rajamma told us that initially there was resistance from the community but the Regis, along with their small group of trained women, gradually won the villagers over.

In 2010, when I was there, the twenty-four-bed THI hospital at Sittilingi with its neonatal ward, operation theatre (OT) and special TB Unit, covered over 10,000 families spread across 20 km. Around 200 births took place at the institution every year. OPD was held thrice a week, with a daily attendance of 150–160 patients. In the OT, lit by a single bulb and equipped with a World War II air and ether anaesthesia kit, non-blood surgeries were carried out. The user fee for tribals was Rs 20 and for non-tribals, Rs 30. In-patients paid whatever they could afford. The results of the THI were, we learnt, astounding. The infant mortality rate had reduced from 150 per 1000 live births to twenty. Consequently, family size had come down to four or five. There had been no maternal deaths in eight consecutive years.

'Over time, we realized that just providing health care wasn't enough. We did a *padayatra* (foot march) in our villages to ask people what they wanted. Their major worry was livelihoods. Second was the issue of younger people migrating. Farming was the main occupation so we introduced organic cultivation. A cooperative of 200 farmers was formed. They grow organic turmeric, cotton, sugarcane and millets. Women make ragi papad and biscuits, and sell them under the brand name Svad,' Regi informed us.

Once, during a field visit, Lalitha discovered the Lambada embroidery done by the women. The art was dying and only two women in the community still knew how to embroider. Lalitha encouraged them and offered to sell their work. These two women trained others and, today, they create beautiful organic and handwoven skirts, tops, bags and so on, under the brand name 'Porgai', meaning pride. These sell at exhibitions in metros. 'Last year, we sold products worth Rs 3 lakh,' Lalitha told us.

In their efforts to transform the community in Sittilingi, the Regis were aided by a few friends. Krishna was one such person. An architect by profession, he designed the Sittilingi hospital using local materials instead of an antiseptic, impersonal building. The result was a house of health where patients feel at ease. After the building was done, Krishna did not leave. Instead, he started training fourteen- to eighteen-year-olds to become entrepreneurs. 'The dropout rate after Class 8 is high as children go to work at the knitwear units in Tirupur. So, we have introduced a one-year academic and technical training course for such boys. I have taught them plumbing, electric works, etc. We have now trained a total of twenty-five students,' Krishna told us.

Speaking to these dedicated doctors, we understood the difficulty of replicating and upscaling these models. In a country where doctors are willing to pay huge amounts of money to escape rural postings, finding practitioners who are willing to stay in tribal hamlets and treat the people is difficult. The exceptions are the Regis or the Jan Swasthya Sahyog of Ganiyari or the Bangs of Gadchiroli. The danger that hangs over such well-meaning initiatives is the challenge to ensure that they can carry on even in the absence of their founding members—a daunting task. We left Sittilingi with the hope these professionals would be able to inspire medical graduates to fulfil their Hippocratic Oath. Today, THI has a team of over seventy highly trained people working to improve the lives of the tribal communities living in the Sittilingi valley and surrounding hills, so our wish is being fulfilled.

EHSAAS: Solan, Himachal

I would like to end this piece with a single person's initiative in Anech village, in the Solan district of Himachal Pradesh. EHSAAS

(Enacting Health and Social Awareness Among the Struggling) is an intervention that targets migrant labour. It is based in Dagshai, next to the better known Sabattu Cantonment and Kasuali.

This is the single-person effort of Ahmed Zaheer, a highly successful dermatologist, who was once affiliated with high specialty hospitals of Delhi. My visit was to find out what made him withdraw from a roaring practice and identify this small village as his 'karmabhoomi'. No government intervention had reached here in thirty years since a real-estate developer discovered its scenic location and brought migrant labourers from Nepal and the tribal areas of Jharkhand to construct holiday homes in the area.

I visited EHSAAS in 2020, six years after I had completed my Planning Commission term. There I met Dr Ahmed. 'One word that sums up my commitment is *ehsaas*, a word which means awareness, and which is the anagram for this intervention,' he said, explaining his philosophy to me, which stems from his belief that prayer is not only observing rituals but also offering service to humanity. He quoted the Sufi poet Shaikh Saadi:

> *Ibadat ba juz khidmat e khalq neest*
> *Ba tashbih o sajjadah o dalq neest*

> Without the service of humanity, prayer means nothing
> It is not counting beads, sitting on the mat
> Or wearing tatters

Over a four-year period, EHSAAS has concentrated on children's health, treatment of anemia and skin infections—bacterial, boils, fungus. The initiative has gone beyond treatment to raising hygiene awareness among families. Voluntary teachers from nearby villages impart general knowledge, respect for each other's religious beliefs and encourage sports and extracurricular activities.

'Getting the smiles back on the faces of families in a remote corner of Solan district is my reward,' Dr Ahmed said as I was leaving.

* * *

I conclude with this small four-year-old experiment because it is an example of a single person making a difference in a small area—a possibility that exists for anyone who feels the compulsion to make a difference. My ancestor, Khwaja Abdullah, patron saint of Herat (then part of greater Iran), wrote at the start of the eleventh century:

> *The world is a mere crossing*
> *And not an abiding city of delight*

This realization is our imperative to give and give, even if it is in a small way.

Co-producing and Pluralizing Health Knowledge for Re-visioning Development

Ritu Priya

Introduction

The past century has seen tremendous gains in the health of Indians, with doubling of life expectancy from about thirty-five years in 1950 to nearly seventy years in 2019. Significant declines have occurred in maternal and child mortality, undernutrition and communicable diseases. This is evidence of the benefits of overall social and economic development, including health services, which have led to an improved quality of life for a significant proportion of the population.

How can we build on these gains of the twentieth century in the most optimal way? Simultaneously, we must acknowledge the challenges we face in the twenty-first century in ensuring continuing improvements in health.

There are fallouts of the past and present path of development. That high-income countries are facing stagnation of life expectancies and even decline in some years gives food for thought.[1] Challenges have been created by encroachments on nature's balances, environmental degradation and pollution, escalating income and asset inequalities, rising income insecurities, nutritional imbalances, rising social conflict and violence, weakening of community social support structures, decline of public services in health and rising costs of health care. The colonial, consumerist economic growth model of development of the nineteenth and twentieth centuries, accentuated by corporate globalization since the 1990s, has much to answer for in this context.

This essay studies the story of Acute Encephalitis Syndrome (AES) in Gorakhpur to illustrate the complexity of issues facing public health today. Extrapolating from it, this piece builds an understanding of the landscape of contemporary India and its implications for health and health care. Ignoring the complexity of public health challenges has been recognized as a reductionist approach to development and sustainable solutions need to be designed as feasible pathways. The essay presents a framework to make it possible to address such issues in all their complexity. For this, I argue that context-sensitive and bottom-up perspectives for systems development are necessary. This would require 'co-producing knowledge' with the relevant actors and segments of society, decolonizing our minds to think in ways specific to the Indian context; and building flexibility for integrating plural approaches within the system. This will mean dealing with the power equations that constitute the politics of knowledge that underlies the health crisis today.

Lessons from AES and Child Deaths in Gorakhpur

In India, childhood illnesses peak annually between June and October, with paediatric wards overflowing and a high number of deaths in district hospitals across the country. These are a result of the malnutrition, water-related and vector-borne diseases that are highest in these pre-harvest and rainy months. Among the infectious diseases causing child deaths, one that has been prominently highlighted in the popular media is Acute Encephalitis Syndrome

(AES) in Gorakhpur district, with the blame being laid at the door of the public medical college hospital and its facilities and doctors.

In Gorakhpur, the peaks are during July–August. Despite being a recognized phenomenon since the 1970s, AES continues to be called *'navki bimari'* (new disease) in local parlance. The perception that these child deaths are not explainable by any single known cause, or effectively prevented despite intensive efforts, makes it a continuing mystery.

The History

Over the early 1970s, the government medical college in Gorakhpur started getting more and more cases of young children with fever, convulsions and loss of consciousness— signs of some sort of encephalitis (i.e., inflammation of the brain tissue). However, there was no understanding of what the killer disease was. In 1978, Dr Kushwaha of the Department of Paediatrics of the public medical college first identified the 'mysterious' disease that was causing child deaths in the area as Japanese Encephalitis (JE), a viral disease spread by mosquito bite. Initially this diagnosis was not accepted and he had to fight many battles to get facilities for the hospital and save the lives of children, generally of poor families who are brought in a serious condition after having been treated by a range of private practitioners. Over the years, the central and state governments have increased the facilities for treatment of AES patients in the medical college, with a special ward and ICU being created in the medical college and the district hospital. After a huge outbreak in 2005, the government started to vaccinate all the children in the region against JE.

A special unit of the National Institute of Virology (Pune) was also opened to study the problem in depth. Studies by the unit have found that besides JE, enteroviruses (spread through contaminated water) and scrub typhus (caused by a bacterium spread by the bite of mites thriving in damp conditions) were causing the encephalitis.[2] Since all of them have similar symptoms affecting the brain, they together form the Acute Encephalitis Syndrome (AES) in the region. All three are water-related infections.

AES has no specific treatment except anti-convulsant medicines, oxygen and keeping respiration going while the body's natural defence mechanisms work to deal with the infection. Under ICMR guidelines, antibiotics that work against scrub typhus are now given to all children with AES. Public ambulances, provided free of charge on call, are functional, with staff trained for handling AES cases. Reportedly, JE cases have reduced, whether due to vaccination or the shift in diagnosis to scrub typhus and enteroviruses is difficult to say. Case fatality of AES has also come down to some extent.[3]

A Complex Story

After a particularly bad incident of oxygen shortage was highlighted in the media as leading to excess AES deaths in August 2017,[4] I visited Gorakhpur in December 2017 to study the situation. I found that the health services were delivering what medical technology could within the constraints of funds and personnel. With a high inflow of patients, doctors and nurses were trying their best, knowing full well that whatever they did, about one-third of the children would die.

Obviously, the causes for child deaths went beyond hospital management issues to those of poverty, malnutrition and the lack of easy access to primary and secondary-level services, so that children came to the hospital late and in a serious condition. However, the adverse media attention resulted in suspensions and arrests of doctors and other staff. The public system had taken another beating in the public eye, adding to the ongoing drift towards the private sector for health care.

Health Care at the Periphery: A Mutual Distrust

National guidelines for management of AES at primary, secondary and tertiary levels show that most cases need not go to a tertiary centre. The government has set up Encephalitis Treatment Centres in over a hundred Primary Health Centres and Community Health Centres in Gorakhpur and adjoining districts. A room exclusively meant to treat AES cases, with oxygen cylinders, anti-convulsant medicines and antibiotics is present at each health centre.

What a doctor at a PHC told us is instructive: 'My first concern is my safety, so how can I treat a child with encephalitis here? If the child dies, the local politicians will lead a mob to lynch me.' The residences for doctors are leaking and ill-maintained; they do not stay there. The women we met in a village spoke of how all staff in the PHC insist on being 'paid', few medicines are available and ASHA workers divert patients referred to the District Hospital to private nursing homes. So why should they go to the PHC at all? This situation of mutual distrust is a fatal flaw for the system's performance.

Instead of resolving the inadequacies of the system that create conflict between doctors and the public at the periphery, the solution is sought in more centralized, expensive, tertiary facilities. The medical college hospital had over 280 paediatric beds. Another 500 paediatric beds have since been added there, an All-India Institute of Medical Sciences (AIIMS) has been built in Gorakhpur, and the Gorakhdham Ashram has built its own super-speciality hospital. But even as wards are added, they fall short, since Gorakhpur is perceived as the only centre for treatment of AES in a 300 km radius. So sick children travelling for long distances to get to Gorakhpur, are denied the timely treatment that could have saved them if trustworthy primary- and secondary-level facilities had been available closer home.

Non-Medical Prevention Missing: Ecosystem Effects

AES patients come to Gorakhpur from rural, urban and peri-urban areas in a 300 km radius. The geography of the region—which is located in the *terai* of the Himalayas, is intersected by rivers, and gets heavy water flow and rainfall during the monsoon— leads to water accumulations and damp conditions. Development of embankments and roads further compounds the problem by blocking natural drainage channels. Flooding has increased to the extent that area under *kharif* crops has reduced to almost one-third. No wonder then that vector and water-borne diseases—including AES—abound, together with malnutrition.

However, the same model of infrastructure development continues with greater vigour. The drainage of the area, including in the city and the hospital, is in a sad state. High-rise residential complexes are coming up in new parts of the city, emulating those in metropolises such as Mumbai and Delhi, despite the fact that before their foundations can be laid, underground water has to be pumped out for weeks. This water is channelled to the city's peri-urban areas. Anecdotal evidence says that AES cases are increasing in Gorakhpur's peri-urban area.

These ecosystem conditions raise the question: can the problem of AES be tackled in the region by merely adding more hospitals and paediatric beds and by making primary and secondary care more community-friendly to decongest the overflowing wards, or is an alternative, healthier model of urban and regional planning simultaneously necessary to stem the flow of cases?

This is a question that is applicable to all of health-care planning across the country.

Implications for the Indian Landscape: Planning Beyond the Rural–Urban Binary

The Indian landscape has been viewed as a binary of rural and urban areas in development planning. Urban areas are viewed as the 'engines of economic growth' and all planning for the future assumes that increasing urbanization is the way to go. Despite this, in 2018, about 65 per cent of Indians still lived in rural areas, and over 50 per cent were engaged in agriculture and allied activities. While data indicates that 35 per cent of India's population lives in urban areas, the 2011 census showed us that the result of rapid urbanization was partly due to over 2500 villages being added as new 'census towns' after 2001. These were categorized as such on the basis of having a population of over 5000 persons, a population density of over 400 persons per sq. km and 75 per cent of working males not employed in agriculture.[5] But these 'towns' still have about 25 per cent residents in agriculture and have low infrastructure development, thereby remaining semi-rural. Similarly, the ribbon development of infrastructure along highways and certain regions in urban areas as well as the continuing of agriculture and allied activities within pockets in urban areas creates peri-urban spaces that reflect a mix of urban and rural characteristics. While data is not collected for what percentage of the population lives under semi-rural and peri-urban conditions, it is evident that a substantial proportion on both sides of the rural–urban binary would fall within them. With even our metropolises being interspersed with areas of agriculture, animal husbandry and fishing, the reality of a continuum of peri-urban, urban, rural and semi-rural agricultural landscape raises the question: are these spaces of transition and bridging between the rural and urban an obsolete remnant to be cast off to create our Smart Cities, or an advantage for resilient and sustainable development, including urbanization?

The binary of town and countryside and the image of the pristine, imperial cities that the Euro-American model of development of the nineteenth and twentieth centuries has given the world precludes recognition of the rural-semirural-peri-urban-urban continuum. We keep attempting to fit ourselves into this binary while our reality is very different, as in other low- and middle-income countries.[6] We have a Town and Country Planning Organization, but even our biggest metropolises and most planned cities such as Delhi and Mumbai remain a mix of 'rural' and 'urban' characteristics. Since we do not plan for the continuum, we are only catering formal services to a fraction of the city's population, with about half to one-third getting access to safe water supply, sewage connections and formally developed residential areas. Transport, industry and dense human populations add to air, soil and water pollution at a rate that the environment is not able to decontaminate, and it seeps into our food chains as well, affecting human and animal health. Meanwhile, the peri-urban and rural suffer the consequences of unbridled urban consumption of resources and environmental degradation caused beyond the urban boundaries.

With our governance systems working with the binary view, assets such as agricultural land are taken up for 'public purposes' with negligible monetary compensation for the original villagers. Once a peri-urban village becomes part of the municipal boundary of a town or city, it ceases to have the panchayat system and thus the support it offers for agricultural activities. The primary health care services offered to rural populations too disappear. Municipal services such as piped water supply and sewage or drainage are generally short even for the city's core areas; such additional peripheries of the city often do not get them at all. Further, they tend to suffer the pollution generated by industrial units, the city's solid waste dumps, sewage and waste water treatment plants that tend to be located in these parts. Participatory governance structures and primary health services are weaker in urban areas and so, in sum, the residents of the peri-urban areas suffer a net loss rather than gain in quality of life and health, despite more cash in hand.[7]

Studies have shown the value of peri-urban and urban agriculture for alleviating urban poverty, providing locally produced perishable items such as leafy vegetables to urban populations, improving urban environments by remediation with cultivation of de-polluting plant species, reducing heat island effects, and providing a creative relationship between nature and human communities, thereby contributing to building of health-care habitats[8, 9]—which foster healthy living and working places for people. Animal husbandry in peri-urban areas again provides perishables such as milk and meat. It also makes possible the agro-ecological relationship of courtyard manure and organic farming. It provided resilience during the COVID-19 pandemic and can mitigate the ravages of climate change. Thus, acknowledging the continuum would add value to urban life in multiple ways, apart from improving health and wellbeing in and beyond the urban habitats.

However, it would require major shifts in thinking; instead of urban and rural planning, we would have to undertake regional planning. Land use planning, such as living and workspaces, will have to be undertaken with considerations of health and equity. The densely populated urban areas and the greener and open peri-urban areas with urban 'sprawl' will need to be co-planned, with context-specific consideration of their epidemiological and management needs.

Urban planning as a modern discipline was initiated in response to the communicable disease epidemics and malnutrition in the post-Industrial Revolution cities of Europe in the nineteenth century. A Delhi or a Mumbai trying to imitate a London or a New York, or Gorakhpur trying to emulate the same architecture, is neither a sustainable enterprise nor does it ensure the wellbeing of its residents. Reimagining our 'urban spaces' with more context-suited rather than colonial lenses requires bottom-up perspectives. Solutions that people have informally evolved to improve their life conditions must be understood and examined for planning more liveable and healthy cities.[10, 11] The models adopted would have to provide multiple approaches with a pluralist framework rather than a one-size-fits-all approach.

A Framework for Unravelling the Complex Crisis of Health-Care Systems

This need for decolonizing, co-producing and pluralizing development approaches applies to other dimensions of health and health care as well. Here is a framework to enable greater understanding of the complexity of health care, provide solutions, enhance health-promoting activities and design effective health services.

State, Market, Professionals, Civil Society, Communities and the Politics of Knowledge

The present crisis in health care has multiple dimensions. The two most commonly identified are the inequities in distribution of health resources and low fund allocation to health service systems by the state. Viewing this merely as an economic and financing issue, however, may not be enough to deal with the health-care crisis. This section will focus on what is often ignored in analyses of the health system and its inequities: the politics of knowledge that underlies the shaping of health care in any society.

The state, market, professional expertise, civil society and communities are five actors that play a role in shaping the health system. The state engages in health systems design and implementation at the formal level. However, an equal or even larger segment of health action forms various kinds of informal health care. Together, the formal and informal interact and form the actual real-life societal 'health system'. While the state implicates national boundaries, international dynamics influence the national and sub-national shaping of health care. Shaping of formal health systems design and the informal health care are both societal processes, with economic, cultural, political, scientific, technological and administrative factors interacting in shaping this dynamic phenomenon.

The complex, non-linear relationships across these five actors can be analysed in some detail by breaking them down into three underlying processes:

- the nature of knowledge/understanding that shapes the design of health service systems, governance structures and policies, and the interaction of formal systems with informal community processes,

- the nature of governance, i.e., the principles and values on which societal decisions are to be made and the structures for doing so, and,
- the distribution of resources across the various social segments, which determines their health status and their ability to access health care.

In this section, we focus on the significance of the first, i.e., the role of the politics of knowledge in the linkage between health systems design, governance, and the access to health resources of the various social segments.

Figure1: Conceptualizing Health Systems Design Holistically: A Framework for Understanding Health Systems Processes and the Politics of Knowledge

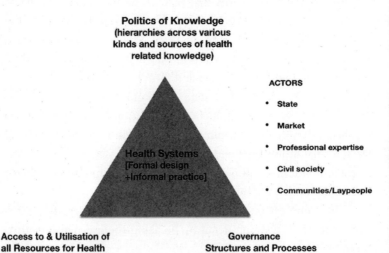

While the international and national economics of health care, shaped by the medical industrial complex with its commercial and professional interests, is a prominent factor in medical and health care systems design; it too works through generating 'knowledge' or 'evidence' that furthers its interests by influencing medical practice and health policy. Civil society, community and lay people's knowledge is axiomatically shaped by ground realities and contextual practices geared to people's interests. Caught in between the commercial interests of the medical industrial complex and the social realities of people's health, are health-care providers who are trained in the former dominant knowledge frame (informed by the medical industrial complex) but wish to ethically apply medical science without being part of its exploitative dimensions. Other health providers, exposed to other knowledge traditions, and appreciative of their value for people's health interests, attempt to make rational sense for plural integrative practice. Thus, what plays out in systems design, policy and practice is the balance of power between the various sources and kinds of health knowledge. This is the 'politics of knowledge' that is evident in our health-care system, composed of its formal and 'informal' components.

'Politics' refers here to the equations of unequal power and processes emanating from it. The power play is evident in which kind of knowledge generation is supported by the state and the market, thereby getting formal legitimacy and playing a dominant role in the formal institutional processes of governance and policy framing, for instance the medical-clinical experts who supervene over public health expertise, or social science knowledge of health that gives an understanding of the diversity of people's health knowledge, perceptions and experiences. Thus, the politics of knowledge and governance result in the choice of a health system design, which in turn influences the access and utilization of services by various social strata. The ground reality of access to various health resources by different communities and sections of society, along with their socially acquired understanding of health issues, leads to their health-seeking behaviour and utilization of services. This in turn influences the designing of the health system, and composes the informal part of the health system.

The issue of 'access' points to the inequity in basic needs fulfilment, including food, housing, water, sanitation and education, among others. The lack of free quality health services in a situation of low purchasing power leads to poor access to health care for many Indians. It is well understood that low purchasing power is related to the social structure, with caste, class and gender interacting to create a certain historically determined inequality frame. Despite decades of post-Independence development, it has been difficult to break this social stratification, though cracks have certainly been made and a better base achieved for standard of living of all. On the other hand, degradation of ecosystems and loss of community control over natural resources has limited their access, causing loss of livelihoods, adequate diversified diets and raw materials of traditional medicine.

Access and the Politics of Knowledge

Health problems of various social segments vary and whose concerns get priority attention and funding in health policy and services development and the research underlying it is one of the primary ways by which the politics of access plays out. This links access to the politics of knowledge. Access is also related to the structure of the health-care system, and that is built on the understanding about health care. Which knowledge framing dominates in the societal shaping of health care depends on the 'politics of knowledge'.

Whether the narrow understanding of health care as 'medical services' (which is what reflects the priority of the better off who have basic needs well met) is used or the wider attention to healthy environment and social structuring for a healthy people (as greater priority for the health of the poorer sections) is one example from within contemporary health sciences that affects policy processes directly. Also, if wider understanding is adopted it will benefit all sections; the trade-off will be with profiteering of the medical industrial complex and unsustainable socio-economic development.

There is secondly, the politics of knowledge in the world of health research, the development of health technologies, of guidelines by expert groups for specific diseases, and advocacy for their adoption through health systems research and publication. This has the medical industrial complex play its very central role, with conflicts of interest between the health benefit to patients/ people versus over-medicalization and the profits accruing from it.

Placing value on the patients' knowledge about their own bodies and its changes, together with that of the doctor or health-care provider's as expert knowledge, is a third dimension of the politics of knowledge. On the one hand, it can lead to a more satisfactory doctor–patient interaction, effective utilization and, on the other, facilitate more rational self-care and agency of people. When lay knowledge is not valued, the health-care provider need not listen to the patient beyond her primary complaint.

Further, this devaluing of human experience extends to replacing the doctor's human clinical skills with a battery of tests rather than using them merely as aids to clinical skills. This precludes the health-care provider's experience-based intuitive capacities to diagnose and treat and is a fourth dimension. 'Evidence-based medicine' that relies only on clinical trials that are carried out under a certain set of conditions and clinical decisions taken according to a specified protocol may not be applicable to all contexts or all kinds of patients but has become the widely accepted best practice. A 'practitioner-based experiential knowledge' that uses the 'evidence-based' protocol but combines it with local variations, individual variations and experience of what works for whom and when has been found to be more effective in real life.[12]

The hierarchy of health knowledge systems or what is often called 'medical pluralism' displays a sixth example of politics of knowledge, where conventional biomedicine is considered the supreme and foremost knowledge, with even the other textual systems that have received state recognition being delegitimized— for instance in India these are Ayurveda, Yoga and Naturopathy, Unani, Siddha, Sowa-Rigpa and Homoeopathy (with AYUSH as the official acronym). The reference point for their validation has become bio-medical science. This denies the validity of diverse ways of viewing the body, its health and disease, thereby losing out on the rich complementarity of perspectives and practices. Even lower in the hierarchy is the knowledge of traditional healers who are not graduates of the formal AYUSH colleges and the home remedies that constitute local health traditions (LHT). While people practise pluralism, that is use more than one knowledge system for various health needs, and WHO recognizes the fact of its widespread practise across all countries,[13] WHO's own health systems framework does not give these knowledge traditions any space.[14] This creation of silos of formal systems knowledge and other knowledges creates a sub-optimal system that favours unnecessary and expensive medicalization at the cost of people's wellbeing. The other knowledges suffer a decline, and people, especially the poorer sections, tend to lose out on access to what earlier was sustainable health care.

While health is a physical and psychological experience, it is also an embodiment of the social situation of a person or sub-group.[15] A patient/people-centred approach requires understanding all these dimensions. However, the social science contributions in health studies, that help us understand the social processes that affect health, tend to be much lower in the hierarchy relative to the medical clinical and technological sciences. This is a seventh dimension of the politics of knowledge that works to the detriment of creating people-centred health care.

All these hierarchies within the realm of knowledge have been generated by institutional processes of legitimization and knowledge management of the colonial and post-colonial state, through its processes of governance. They continue to be actively supported by the global and national medical industrial complex. As these contemporary institutional processes penetrate the AYUSH systems, the medical industrial complex enhances its profits through them too, and reduces even their comprehensiveness, eco-friendly and sustainable characteristics.[16]

Governance and the Politics of Knowledge

Governance on a societal scale is what the state agencies construct. As societal arbiters, they decide which knowledge and whose knowledge is to be used to shape policy approaches and health care. How much centrality is given to the medical industrial complex and the markets it generates, and how much to a pro-people, bottom-up perspective is a vital element of governance. The welfare state was meant to bring both together by taking the benefits of modern science and technology to the masses, the state being the financier and provider of services. This has democratized the access to health-care resources in terms of universal entitlements for all. However, this remains a principle that is denied in practice by the dominance of the social elite combined with the colonial flow of health knowledge continuing into postcolonial times. The bureaucracy and its methods for population-level systems development tend to find it convenient to draw from the global health knowledge system and ignore the informal component of the grounded realities of health care. This has led to a top-down techno-managerial approach to dominate the policy frame rather than a social structural and bottom-up approach. The technocratic dominance of governance received a further fillip through the use of ICT and big data analytics in tandem with insurance systems and the bio-technology industry. This was abundantly observed during the COVID-19 pandemic as well.[17]

Civil society actors and social movements have been at the forefront of highlighting the social dimensions of health in public discourse. Public health academics and professionals who have adopted more holistic theoretical approaches have been an active stream of expertise that is different from the contemporary dominant mainstream knowledge frame. They have pioneered shifts in thinking about health care and health systems development over the years, or about clinical practice, or technology development. And many of the shifts have come about by 'learning from the people'. Jenner's development of the smallpox vaccine, the development of Oral Rehydration Solution for diarrhoeal disease, the development of pharmaceutical products extracted from traditional herbal medicines, are among the many examples of this. The Alma Ata declaration stating the Primary Health Care approach was also an outcome of such a people-empowering orientation.[18]

Communities of lay people, in living their daily lives and handling health problems, have most often been the repositories and filters of what works and what does not for them, in their conditions of constraints and opportunities. They draw from all possible sources that which seems to work, whether it is from their informal socialization and cultural context as traditional knowledge and practices, or their education by formal systems and service providers. As they adapt to changing situations and needs, they weigh the costs and benefits. What gets incorporated at a community or societal level is thus patterns of health-care and health-seeking behaviours that they consider most suited to their context.

Rejection of prescribed medical interventions, or 'default', may sometimes turn out to be rational decisions taken under real-life conditions, and several studies have verified this.[19, 20] Thereby, improving the conditions of life such that the most health-generating behaviours become the most naturally rational, rather than 'victim blaming', is a critical approach in public health. The continuing utilization of traditional medical systems, and increasing resort to them too, must be viewed in this light of experiential rationality.

People of all social segments have common elements in the health care that they aspire to. For instance, all would want their doctor or health-care provider to consider them rational human beings and treat them with dignity, listen seriously to their understanding of their health problems, give them additional information they do not have and advise them based on the best knowledge the health system has at its command. All they want is that this process be driven by considerations of their wellbeing and not commercial interest.

However, studies also show that the perceived source of individual wellbeing, dignity and health is influenced by the collective social identity. While an expensive stay at a private hospital may be perceived by the rich as something that gets them greater prestige in their community, women being given a role in taking decisions about themselves and their health has been important for the women's movement since the 1970s. Dalit groups identify with it in terms of getting out of the practice of untouchability and other traditional forms of discrimination, such as bans on their consumption of status goods. Thus, accessing modern health care is a component of their sense of dignity in the present times. Cultural identity assertion, with its closeness to forest and nature, is central to the Adivasi's sense of community dignity, and thereby they assert their traditional health practices as well. All this social diversity of perceptions influences health-seeking behaviours and their degree of trust in the health system.[21]

Non-understanding of this social and cultural context and an overwhelming influence of the medical industrial complex on governance, health systems design and the practice of health services has generated a mutual distrust between the people and the health service system. This is where the politics of knowledge and the political economy of health care needs to be addressed, with the processes of decolonization, co-production and pluralizing of the knowledge framework for health-care policy, planning and practice, re-orienting the design of the health-care system.

Conclusion: Addressing Contextual Realities, Creating Health-Care Habitats

This essay proposes that we need to reconceptualize our systems and how we plan for them—for instance, the urban spaces and our health system. It proposes the adoption of an ecological and social approach to health care and public health. It calls for a shift in the 'politics of knowledge' towards a more holistic, context-sensitive approach than the currently dominant technology-oriented, over-medicalized and globally prescribed models. Such an approach is not posed as an either-or but as a systemic mode that views the formal and informal components as an integral whole. It would then holistically provide for better health and wellbeing, with decentralized and pluralist approaches. The essay suggests that the big innovation required is in terms of how a shift in mindset is to be brought about at societal scale. It includes broad basing the involvement of actors engaged in designing and implementing health-care systems at all levels through a dialogic mode. A framework that gives one an understanding of the complex processes underlying and shaping the formal and informal components of the health system has been suggested. The dynamics of power hierarchies of three major phenomena—the knowledge sphere, governance and access—involve interactions of the state, market, professionals, civil society and communities. Addressing these through an understanding of the politics of knowledge will benefit not only the informal, but also make the formal system more realistic and effective.

The ecological crisis and the COVID pandemic have generated a wider recognition of the need for such a shift. The UN's seventeen SDGs provide an opportunity for such a shift but sustainable development has to be implemented with greater synergy between these goals and with addressing of issues of the marginalized sections.

A mindset shift under SDG 11 (stated to 'Make cities and human settlements inclusive, safe, resilient and sustainable') would involve consideration of what the urban spaces in India represent, what is their relationship with the larger whole including the rural, their diversity across the country and in their social structure, and therefore how their development should be envisaged. It suggests, for instance, creating Health-Care Habitats across the rural-semirural-peri-urban-urban continuum of the Indian landscape. This approach would consider implications of all development activities on the ecosystem and infrastructure, livelihoods and basic needs, social relations, social services especially facilities for health of children, women and the elderly, and meaningful engagement in collective activities to fulfil higher order/spiritual needs of all for better health and wellbeing.

This would require macroeconomic structural planning to factor in the optimal role of various sectors of the economy from the perspective of the rural-urban continuum and all sections of the population. Urban design that ensures healthy flows of water and waste will need context-sensitive planning. Regional land-use planning has to ensure clustered multi-purpose activities crossing the rural–urban divide such that work spaces and residential spaces make for liveable habitats. Providing green spaces of various types that ensure an optimal mix of green livelihood options, outdoor exercise and leisure activities, will require innovative regional and urban planning, combining compact urban construction and a peri-urban/rural sprawl. Agro-ecological zones can fulfil these desirables in and around cities, and in addition add to food availability and contribute to mitigating environmental degradation.

Similarly, a more democratic ethos that acknowledges the rationality of people's perspectives can lead to doctor–patient interactions respectful of the patient's knowledge and experience, and to integrating diverse knowledges at various levels of the health-care system. The diversity of people's health-care practices, experiences and priorities would help inform what the health-care system should optimally be like. Collective health-care decisions based on bottom-up processes of context-specific need assessment, decentralized planning and contextualized policy formulation in collaboration with the best in practice-based evidence and public health expertise should become the mode of governance. The health services component of Health-Care Habitats per se should be designed with a decolonized mindset, based on co-production of knowledge; addressing health disparities from their socio-economic correlates and the pluralistic cultural dimensions of health care. Then all Indians will be able to live healthier lives, with conditions that contribute to social cohesion, greater confidence and ownership in a caring state and trust in health-care systems.

Creating a System of Health-Care Providers for Universal Health Coverage

K. Sujatha Rao

Tracing History

Memories of visiting my uncle during the 1950s and '60s, in the small village of Arugolanu, about 40 km from Vijayawada, are still fresh in my mind. He was a licentiate doctor (LIM), who graduated from the School of Indian Medicine that was affiliated to the Madras Medical College. The LIM or the Licentiate in Integrated Medicine was a five-year course where the students were trained in Ayurveda, Unani, Siddha, and for two years in allopathy. Instituted in 1923, the course had a separate registration since 1933. The LIM graduates were expected to work in rural areas and were eligible to be employed by local boards.

My uncle owned vast stretches of land that served as his main source of income. He was the only doctor for 15 miles around. He treated all ailments—coughs, fevers, body pains, first aid for injuries, snake bites and so on—besides proficiently conducting deliveries. He also worked in the District Board's dispensary for a monthly salary of Rs 200 or so.

Riding in his horse buggy with his brown leather bag in hand, which contained medicines, a stethoscope, a BP-measuring equipment, bandages and such sundry materials, my uncle would attend to house calls, day or night. Keeping vigil over a critical patient and returning home in the wee hours of morning was normal. He knew his patients by name and remembered their medical histories. He was respected and popular, and trading his power to heal for cash was never a consideration. As the family doctor, he felt morally responsible for the wellbeing of his patients, in turn, earning their gratitude. Then, medical treatment was all about trust and social relationships, a far cry from what we witness today.

There were several classes of medical doctors in the Madras Presidency. The vaids and hakims were at the bottom. Layered above were the LIMs, the three-year allopathy-trained Licentiates of Medical Practice (LMP) and the MBBS graduates. The latter two worked in government hospitals occupying the posts of surgeons, civil assistant surgeons and assistant surgeons. Such non-standardization of provider skills was to make the provisioning of rural health services affordable.[1] However, the LMPs always smarted under this system as they felt more like 'glorified ward boys or qualified quacks'.[2] They demanded parity with the MBBS doctors to improve their career prospects. In 1938, the Madras Presidency abolished the LMPs by increasing the course duration from three to five years. By 1947 when India won independence, there were 29,870 LMPs and 17,654 MBBS doctors.

The 1943 Health Survey and Development Committee, chaired by Sir Joseph Bhore as its Chairman, submitted its report in 1946. It provided the whole architecture for delivering services at decentralized levels that holds good even for today. The report's recommendations sought to replace the low-cost LMP system by the more expensive District Health Organization (DHO), consisting of one Primary Health Centre, manned by thirty-five persons (two MBBS doctors, a nurse, midwives, public health nurses, laboratory assistant, pharmacist, helpers, etc.) for every 40,000 people, supervised and supported by a seventy-five-bed hospital for every 10,000–20,000 people. The DHO envisaged for secondary care was a 650-bed hospital at a regional level and a 2500-bed hospital at the apex district level.

The financial implications were substantial, necessitating a five-fold increase at a time when India was facing dire challenges of mass hunger, poverty and the problems of partition. In 1948, at the meeting of the Provincial Health Ministers convened to discuss the Joseph Bhore Report on health reform, the importance of Indian systems of medicine and LMPs was asserted. Yet, the drive for modernization and scientific temper led to the abolition of all licentiates. This single decision dealt a body blow to India's attempts to provide a community-based primary health-care system—a blow that we are still to recover from.

Since the implementation of the Bhore Report recommendations was resource intensive, a midway design was developed consisting of block-level Primary Health Centres (PHCs) functioning under the Block Panchayat System. The Primary Health Centres were to be supported by sub-centres for every 10,000 people, manned by an auxiliary nurse midwife (ANM). Alongside were taluk hospitals (coterminous in geographical jurisdiction with block) and district hospitals. In addition were the malaria workers, the traditional birth attendants, sanitary workers, etc. Some were paid employees, while others lived on the fees/contributions of the villagers. The edifice was clearly doctor-centric.

In 1959, the government constituted a committee known as the Health Survey and Planning Committee under the chairmanship of Dr Mudaliar to review the implementation of the Bhore Report. The Mudaliar's Committee Report of 1962[3] recognized that the training imparted made doctors 'more suitable for conditions that prevail in western countries' and not 'relevant' to work in rural conditions. In other words, the doctors appointed to work in

PHCs were ill-prepared to practise in rural settings. The report not only called for more relevant training but also suggested the constitution of an All India Medical Service, like the IAS. Such observations resonated in the reports of several expert committees set up periodically. The Medical Council of India (MCI) paid scant attention to these recommendations that essentially linked training to prevailing health needs whereby the 'basic' doctors are equipped to handle social conditions and be 'social physicians . . . protecting the people and guiding them to good health'.[4] Inappropriate training alienated the doctors from the people, resulting in their frequent absence from work.

Meanwhile, in order to compensate for low salaries, many state governments allowed salaried doctors to practise privately that often meant a private consultation for a fee at the doctors' residences. With time, such private consultations morphed into either owning or consulting in full-fledged nursing homes and hospitals, contributing to the problem of absenteeism with doctors visiting their place of duty only to collect their salaries at worst or attend to a few patients at best. Added to the pull of such strong financial incentives were other factors such as inappropriate accommodation, poor job satisfaction due to non-availability of drugs, diagnostic equipment or infrastructure, a non-conducive social life, and inadequate incentives that exacerbated the problem of chronic absenteeism. This gave rise to the practice referred to as 'doing an up-down'—living in urban towns but working in rural centres. The dichotomy worsened as most doctors belonged to an urbane emerging middle class looking westwards for career progression, instead of wanting to address the basic needs of a people racked by poverty, steeped in superstition and illiteracy.

While at one level, the disparities between rural villages and urban towns were widening, at another level the government also sought to further expand access to primary care by taking facilities closer to the people and also rationalizing the various categories of functionaries in order to bring greater coherence and efficiency in the functioning of the facilities. Accordingly, the Government of India, in 1972, appointed an expert committee under Kartar Singh[5] that recommended the setting up of a Primary Health Centre for every 30,000 people and converting the Block PHC into a thirty-bed Community Health Centre manned by four specialists. Such decentralization, though appropriate, was however no solution in the context of bad weather roads and poor transportation facilities. Since a vacuum cannot remain unfilled for long, over time, the latent demand for basic health services felt at the village/household level was addressed by unqualified quacks. With the abolition of the LMPs and no suitable replacement, compounders and ward boys in doctors' clinics began to proliferate into villages that qualified doctors shunned, treating minor ailments and injuries and calling themselves Rural Medical Practitioners (RMP).

The million-strong RMPs are a poor imitation of the LMPs but enjoy the same level of trust and acceptability from the people, particularly the poor. Living close to them and focusing on services rather than remuneration, they became indispensable. However, a detailed report[6] on Unqualified Medical Practitioners (UMPs) notes that UMP/RMPs, while continuing to be the first point of contact for the poor, have since become 'commission agents' of the increasing number of private nursing homes set up by qualified doctors, getting substantial remuneration for every referral:

> Nursing homes and hospitals need the services of UMPs for getting patients . . . Generous commissions are paid to them by medical establishments. This amounts to a share of around 30 per cent of the fees charged by qualified doctors . . . studies show these earnings account for higher inflows as compared to earnings from providing treatment. This is another pull factor for the UMPs to expand services as they can earn by becoming indispensable to the private medical system.

Human Resource Availability a Key Challenge in Building Primary Health Care

Since the primary health-care structures were to be manned only by a qualified MBBS doctor, their shortage became problematic. Besides, with increasing job opportunities in the US and UK offering three times their earnings in India, the most qualified doctors, trained in public colleges, sought to migrate to greener pastures. In fact, so intense was the brain drain that in 1967, the US ruled that work permits and visas to doctors would mandatorily require a no-objection certificate to be issued by the Government of India.

Notwithstanding the worsening situation of the non-availability of doctors in rural and peri-urban health facilities, public policy response stayed unchanged. Plan after plan, the government had just one solution to the problem of providing health-care services to the people—more and better infrastructure, drugs, equipment and some management training for doctors, without improving and reforming the incentive structures, accountability, outcomes or systems of governance. Despite the increasing politicization and corruption that was adversely impacting the governance of public facilities, discussions related to the poor functioning of the health-care system, revolved around doctor absenteeism or inadequate supply of inputs and infrastructure. Now and again, the suggestion to revive the LMP course as a more advisable strategy would emerge.

After the formation of Chhattisgarh in November 2000, the then Ajit Jogi government approved a three-year medical degree course, aimed at creating a new stream of allopathic practitioners to be deployed to serve in rural areas where MBBS doctors were unwilling to serve. For various reasons ranging from the stiff opposition of the MCI, litigation by the Indian Medical Association (IMA) to issues related to implementation, this innovation was later set aside despite evaluations indicating the doctors' fitness to practise in rural areas being better than that of MBBS graduates[7]. Alongside, a voluntary community health worker scheme, called Mitanin, was launched and tried out. This found its full expression under the National Rural Health Mission of 2005, when the Accredited Social Health Activists (ASHA), located for every 1000 persons in rural areas, was established. The purpose of ASHAs was to connect the people with health-care services, namely immunization and maternal care, gradually expanding to services under communicable and non-communicable disease control programmes. Envisioned as a community representative, ASHAs emerged as the last rung of the health system with a community presence.

In 2018, the government implemented the Ayushman Bharat scheme as a flagship programme. One component of this programme is the strengthening of the sub-centres, renamed as Health & Wellness Centres, which are to be manned by an ANM and a BSc nurse with a six-month public health training qualification—designated as the Mid-Level Health Provider. The Health & Wellness Centres are expected to deliver a package of twelve services, ranging from antenatal to mental health care.

India has a messy health architecture consisting of a four-tiered structure—the medical colleges and hospitals for tertiary care, district and sub-district level hospitals for secondary care, and the CHC-PHC-H&W Centres for primary health care, with ASHAs and Anganwadi Workers at the community level. The key purpose of organizing health services into tiered hierarchies is to enable defining functions and services, skills and competencies to be provided at different levels of care so as to ensure optimizing available resources and rationalizing patient health seeking pathways. But achieving such a purpose requires role clarity and a referral system. In the absence of both, there is much duplication and avoidable inefficiencies. Besides, corresponding to each level of the government structure, there is a similar hierarchy in the private sector, down to the RMPs and practitioners of traditional medicine, with completely different approaches and understandings of health and wellness.

UHC and Human Resources for Health

India has over a million each of doctors, nurses and paramedics and over 7,00,000 AYUSH practitioners. Given the population base, India falls short of achieving the WHO norm of 25.4 health workers per 10,000 persons.[8] Besides, when these statistics are adjusted for quality and geographical unevenness of distribution, the proportion of health workers to persons will fall further. For achieving the global aspiration of Universal Health Coverage (UHC) that is equitable and affordable, the big challenge facing policymakers is designing an appropriate human resources policy.

In keeping with India's aspirations for modernization, the MCI Act of 1956 provided the framework for India's public policy to define what constitutes a basic doctor. By implication, it rejected the existence and validity of other systems of medicine. Paying only a nominal attention to these other systems, public policy aggressively pursued the ambition of creating doctors as good as those available in developed countries. While the nature of training imparted was one that needed more than five years (as the curricula focused both on knowledge as well as skill acquisition), the political pressure to produce doctors within shorter time frames so as to fill up the posts in the facilities being established, compelled a compromise with the quality of education—relaxing norms, reducing course duration, and opening up more colleges despite non-availability of the required faculty. Added to this was the deteriorating fiscal situation that pushed towards private investment. Accordingly, from nineteen medical colleges with 1200 students in 1947, in 2020 there are 612 colleges with 91,927 UG seats: 48,012 in 322 government medical colleges and 43,915 in 290 private medical colleges. The privatization of medical colleges that started in the 1990s accounting for 33 per cent of the 135 medical colleges then, has now increased to 47 per cent.[9]

Though the private sector brought in much-needed investment in medical education in terms of physical infrastructure, it fuelled unbridled commercialization that reduced the objective of medical education to the pursuit of getting dividends and a return on the capital invested rather than the production of well-trained doctors. Quality of instruction became a serious casualty—a fact overlooked by MCI in return for monetary considerations as seen by the several court cases of alleged corruption against the MCI and the scathing 92nd Report of the Parliamentary Standing Committee on the Functioning of the Medical Council of India, 2016. Such privatization also widened regional disparities—origin of investors and students' paying capacity determined the location of the colleges in the economically affluent southern and south-western states. Since the mobility of doctors is dictated by considerations of language, social environment and cultural factors, the non-availability of doctors in the rest of the country was an inevitable consequence. Thirdly, being charged exorbitantly by medical colleges demotivated doctors from working in lesser-paying fields like public health or joining government service to work in rural areas. Instead, doctors sought to either go abroad, work at corporate hospitals where salaries were higher, or set up their own practice in urban areas, thus exacerbating the urban–rural divide.

In keeping with the changing times and a growing awareness of the need for more well-rounded doctors with an awareness of sociology, anthropology, biostatistics and economics, in 2010, the Board of Governors of the MCI held wide consultations to devise a comprehensive curriculum. The proposal provided students choice to opt for public health or a clinical subject after three years of basic training. After eight years, in 2018, some incremental, but much needed, changes were introduced at the MBBS level—information technology, sociology, economics and soft skills, like ethics, attitude, communication with patients in a respectful manner, values and confidentiality incorporated as core attributes in medical professionals.

Current Challenges

The COVID-19 pandemic has once again shifted focus to the importance of containing communicable diseases, as being infectious, they inflict huge damage. Communicable diseases still account for 36 per cent of India's disease burden. Reducing this burden that disproportionately affect the poor, would require revamping health system priorities by increasing focus on public health, family medicine, infectious diseases control programme implementation, etc. The neglect of public health and shift of policy attention towards expanding access to medical treatment of non-communicable diseases has meant the non-availability of critical manpower like epidemiologists, biostatisticians, virologists, immunologists etc. that are required to contain COVID-19 and reduce the burden of disease load in the country. Besides, as the experience of tackling COVID-19 has shown, what is urgently needed is a strong primary health-care system to tackle disease outbreaks at the local level.

A second set of challenges is the dealing with and coopting the technological advances in the field of diagnostics and drugs, resulting in dramatically better outcomes. Artificial intelligence is just round the corner as is personalized medicine. Besides, technology works at all levels. If robots can replace a surgeon in a tertiary hospital, rapid diagnostic tests can replace the laboratory technicians in primary care settings. Increasingly, self-administered diagnostic tests, undertaken in mobile settings with results instantly communicated to remotely located specialists and receiving treatment advice and prescriptions, is emerging as a possible reality, disrupting the manner in which health service delivery systems are currently organized.

Clearly, with the dual burden of disease—one-third communicable and two-thirds non-communicable diseases—India has to be working simultaneously at all levels of health care—finding local solutions aimed at disease prevention and early diagnosis at the primary level and ensuring cure and alleviation of pain and suffering through the intelligent adoption of technology at the tertiary-institutional level. This certainly puts pressure on the health system and on the doctors who are expected to be aware and knowledgeable of the changing scenarios, giving rise to an exponential demand for specialization. The policy response to this changing environment has been to not only increase the number of PG sets but also strengthen the Diplomate of National Board (DNB) process.[10] The DNB is a three-year post graduate course where training is provided by accredited private hospitals and the examination is conducted by the National Board of Examinations—an autonomous academic body established in 1984 under the Ministry of Health and Family Welfare. Today, there are 9796 DNB/FNB courses and 2432 members of the College of Physicians and Surgeons of Mumbai (CPS). Recently, the government overturned the earlier MCI refusal to recognize DNB as an eligibility to apply for faculty posts in some specialties such as obstetrics and gynaecology, paediatrics, family medicine, ophthalmology, ENT, radio diagnosis and TB/chest diseases.

Similar problems of appropriateness of recruitment, duration and quality of training and so on have risen in the context of nurses as well. Technological innovation has thrown up a huge demand for skilled technicians—optometrists, radiology assistants, X-ray technicians, occupational therapists, physiotherapists etc. There is scope for such non-medical personnel to take over several functions hitherto being performed by doctors. For example, today a simple gadget can enable testing eyes at home, screening those necessitating a surgical intervention. Since four-fifths of eye patients need spectacles, this whole spectrum of diagnosis and treatment can be addressed by paramedical professionals, freeing ophthalmologists to attend to surgical correction.

The Future

The health system functions on three prongs: human resources, technology and finances. Doctors—without nurses and paramedical staff, drugs and diagnostics or funds to buy consumables—determine the operational efficiencies of the system. At the core are the medical human resources—their attitudes, training, understandings, perceptions and value systems.

The spectacular failure of the MCI in imparting and regulating a value-based training and ethical practice, and instead getting associated with a 'cash for college and cash for a seat' system inviting scathing indictments from the Supreme Court and the Parliamentary Standing Committee on Health and Family Welfare led to calls for its reform. In 2017, bringing a closure to a process initiated in 2010, the government enacted an alternative to the MCI, renaming it as the National Medical Commission (NCM). This is a thirty-three-member advisory commission with four independent boards: The Under-Graduate Medical Education Board (UGMEB), the Post-Graduate Medical Education Board (PGMEB), the Medical Assessment and Rating Board; and the Ethics and Medical Registration Board.

The NMC Act[11] has two provisions with far-reaching implications for the future direction of the health system: it permits privately managed colleges to levy fees in accordance with market prices for 50 per cent of the student strength and grant limited licence to mid-level practitioners, called *Community Health Providers*, to prescribe medicines for providing primary and preventive health care. Both these provisions are gamechangers. The first will further deepen commercialization, benefiting the investor without contributing to better quality of doctors or patients' wellbeing; the second will empower frontline workers to address people's needs for basic health care.

Medical care is not just about doctors and drugs. It is also about a large number of routine processes, procedures and interventions such as immunization, health education and patient communication for behaviour change. Most diseases are self-limiting or do not become serious if treated adequately and in time. Nurses can be an invaluable resource in undertaking these functions and procedures.

Thus, besides a focus on doctors, there is an equal urgency to make better use of nurses by delegating them routine functions and encouraging task shifting.

Under closer supervision, if provided the skills to undertake abortions, provide family planning services, conduct breech deliveries, diagnose signs of cervix or breast cancer, and treat other women's health issues, graduate nurses would be acceptable and appropriate to a rural India to work as nurse practitioners while at the same time allow doctors to put their long years of arduous training to more optimal use. With the NMC allowing non-medical personnel, such as nurses, working in sub-centres and primary health centres limited powers to prescribe allopathic medicines, there is a huge potential to enhance the optimality of such a cadre of caregivers. Similarly, nurses also have the potential to specialize—in anaesthesia, ICU care, ophthalmology, mental health, operation theatre management, community health etc.

The urgency to focus on a cadre of nurse practitioners needs to be underscored if we want to achieve UHC for essential care in the short and medium term. In the US, nurse practitioners autonomously provide a full range of primary, acute, and specialty health-care services, including ordering, performing and interpreting diagnostic tests such as lab work and X-rays, diagnosing and treating acute and chronic conditions such as diabetes, high blood pressure, infections and injuries, managing patients' overall care and counselling and educating patients on disease prevention and lifestyle choices.

Achieving such a workforce would imply upgrading the skill and knowledge base of nurses, who should be incentivized to complete a master's course, undertake advanced clinical training, and obtain national certification alongside career progression, wider responsibilities and status. Surveys in US and Europe have conclusively shown that nurse practitioners have high patient satisfaction rates, are a cost-effective solution as their early intervention in primary care has resulted in reduced emergency visits, shorter hospital stays and lower medication costs. In cash-strapped economies and with the increasing cost of care, such shifts could have huge fiscal impacts.

Recommendations

Health is a human-resource intensive sector generating direct and indirect employment opportunities. It is also demanding on fiscal resources. The global goal of UHC is to reduce household expenditures to no more than 20 per cent of total health spending. In India, households incur about 69 per cent, due to low public spending, which has stagnated around 1 per cent of the GDP for decades.

While the WHO has defined UHC to imply provisioning of health services as per need through the spectrum of primary to tertiary care in a seamless manner, the Sustainable Development Goals (SDGs) aim to have all countries achieve UHC for essential services at least by 2030. This then provides flexibility for countries to strategize by starting with essential care. So, while Rwanda may define UHC for essential health services to be primary care, UK or Canada could mean all health services with some exceptions like dental. In India, instead of defining UHC in terms of services, it is defined as a population covered under government-sponsored health insurance programmes, which include hospital expenditures incurred on a package of services, combined with the understanding that all primary health care providing essential services are free to all citizens. Financial risk protection for in-patient treatment is, however, restricted to the poor, who constitute 40 per cent of the population.

Achieving the goals of UHC, even in this restricted sense, can be challenging. Following are some recommendations for a way forward:

1. Reverse the policies that are commercializing medical and nursing education. The fees must be affordable and focus

should shift to quality and an admission process where the meritorious and not those with the ability to pay are preferred.

2. Increase public investment to bring medical and nursing colleges up to acceptable standards rather than opening more, except in highly deserving cases. A detailed review of the 'standard' could also help reduce the cost of establishing medical colleges, a reason cited to justify high capitation fees.

3. Instead of being converted into medical colleges, district hospitals should be allowed to enter into long-term MOUs with medical colleges to provide training facilities for their students for a fee determined by the government. This would enable district hospitals to earn a steady stream of revenue that can then be used to improve quality of patient care in their facilities.

4. Revamp the MBBS courses and provide not just a more broad-based and skill-driven curricula but also the choice to take up public health or clinical practice.

5. Accord primacy to public health to reduce the overall burden of infectious and communicable disease and build a comprehensive response plan to be implemented by public health professionals at all levels. For expediting such a revamp, state instrumentalities such as a dedicated Department of Public Health at central and state levels need to be established to enable a comprehensive focus on prevention of disease, promotion and provisioning of basic care in close engagement with communities. In such a public health perspective, ANMs will become community nurses, while professional cadres of Nurse Practitioners, counsellors, nutritionists and biostatisticians will be inducted into the primary health care spectrum. Considering that primary level care accounts for substantial household expenditures incurred on diagnostics and drugs, developing teams of paramedical personnel and nurses at the community level under the guidance of public health physicians trained in Family Health medicine will address 90 per cent of people's

health needs. Well-trained public health teams will also help eliminate unqualified quackery and the cycle of commissions and corrupt practices.

6. As a short-term measure, in health provider-deficit states, reviving the three-year graduate/BSc doctors as rural medical practitioners is justified. To craft such a system, these professionals will need to be trained in medical colleges and district hospitals and registered separately with feasibility for career progression by enabling them to study the additional two years to acquire a MBBS degree. This is a better option than using AYUSH practitioners to prescribe medicines and treatment they are not trained in.

7. A GP- and family doctor-led primary health care system is long overdue. Such a design would imply that a doctor or a team of doctors, public or private, having the requisite infrastructure, acceptable to the people and with capacity to deliver as per standards, are assigned a dedicated population. The difference between the current model and the proposed approach is the shift from facility to doctor. In other words, it is the doctor who is given the 6000 population, that they are then responsible for to ensure the delivery of the guaranteed package of services, referrals, post-hospitalization care, house visits, school health and so on. Payment and incentives will be outcome-based and the doctor, if government-appointed, would be non-transferable for seven years or some such long tenure that will enable measurement of work done. Such a system will shift focus from the PHC as a facility to the doctor and the health teams responsible for population health. Such redesigning would also imply that at the 30-bed Community Health Centres, doctors trained in Family Medicine be posted, to provide the referral and oversight functions over the PHC system. The DNB programme has designed a two-year course in Family Medicine. Making the acquisition of such a degree mandatory for further career progression and allowing paid

study leave for in-service candidates, would help create the required trained manpower in the short/medium term.

8. The district hospitals should act as the gateway to higher levels of care to cater to the 7 per cent of the sick who would need and seek secondary care. It is at this level that specialists in at least fifteen disciplines need to be appointed. Task shifting, by having the surgeons and obstetricians working in district hospitals, to work under the supervision and guidance of a tertiary/super specialty department like oncology or cardiology, could enable building their expertise to take up relatively less complicated surgeries. For example, an obstetrician capable of doing a C-section can as well remove the abdominal tumour of a cancer patient, thereby obviating the need for specialized oncologists to be available in district hospitals, de-clogging the specialty hospitals and enabling a more efficient use of available human resources. Follow-up chemotherapy can likewise be decentralized to district hospitals by providing them with appropriate laboratories and requisite staff. Besides, a further augmentation of human resources at district hospitals can be ensured by posting MD students from medical colleges to work there on a rotation basis. While the students hone up their skills due to the patient load and develop the confidence to perform independently, the patients can also get access to specialist services without having to go to tertiary hospitals.

9. The 2005 National Commission of Macroeconomics and Health Report recommended the standardization of nursing to start with a basic graduate degree as in Thailand. In India there are various levels—10+2 auxiliary nurse midwives (ANM), three-year GNM, four-year trained BSc and so on. With powers to prescribe commonly needed drugs for primary care, well-trained graduate nurses should rapidly become the norm. The ANMs and GNMs can be provided opportunities to study BSc, with course duration adjusted depending on their current level of knowledge and skills.

Besides, the nursing profession needs to have two arms—public health and clinical medicine. The clinical nurses need to be trained in hospital settings and provided avenues for further specialization by way of diplomas to work in specialty clinics. Such separation is critically required so as to avoid nurses being shifted around from ICU management to operation theatres and to rural PHCs. Public health nurses likewise should be provided a choice between becoming nurse practitioners or public health managers, where they carry out administrative jobs. Besides, at the district, state and central level, the head of nursing should be independent and not under the Director of Health or Medical Education for providing focus to the nursing profession that is currently overwhelmed by the demands of medical colleges. In other words, it is critical that the nursing profession be given autonomy and, above all, stature. Finally, the tutors in nursing colleges and nurses working in the field should be transferable so that the tutors stay up to date with the developments and operational issues.

10. Other paramedical personnel such as pharmacists and laboratory technicians and the range of other such personnel working across the cure spectrum need recognition. Recently, the Ministry of Health formulated the 'National Commission for Allied and Healthcare Professions Bill, 2020' to open a registry and build a regulatory system for allied professionals. Besides building a database, it will enable standardization of course curricula, as is already being done in some fields like Physiotherapy, Occupational Therapy, Optometry and Medical Lab Sciences. Such curricula cover Diploma, Bachelors and Postgraduate degrees and provides an understanding of the career options. Further, by being in conformity with global norms, the qualified also gain the advantage of accessing global markets.

In addition to the technical personnel, health also employs a wide range of other professionals to organize and manage the functioning of this complex system of service delivery—janitor to accountants, hospital managers, statisticians, nurses, drivers, cleaners, security, computer software professionals, engineers and so on.

Above all, people and community resources are a vital dimension to the sector. The more the engagement of the community, the better the quality of policy design and effectiveness of implementation. This was best demonstrated in the HIV and AIDS control programme where key population groups, with seven times incidence of HIV infection over general population, were engaged in policy formulation and implementation. Lay persons must be inducted into the NMC and other professional councils, as is the practice in the British Medical Council. This will help the professions stay relevant and need-based and allow people universal access to health care services that they need and deserve, in dignity and a deep sense of solidarity.

This short account of India's health system challenges, with focus on human resources shows the patchy and not coherent public policy to develop a delivery system that is linked to the demand for services, peoples' rapidly changing expectations and behaviour. India is home to multicultural strains of thoughts, ideas and perceptions, besides wide variance of historical legacies and fractured social structures. It is time India crafts policies that are based on the principles of equity, accessibility affordability, sustainability and quality, contextualized to local epidemiological and cultural conditions. Treating the country as a homogenous entity, amenable to one approach was and continues to be an error.

The New Health-Care Paradigm: De-fragmenting Health-Care Systems

Rohina Joshi and Vivekanand Jha

Introduction

India's health system has long been a work in progress, simultaneously dealing with an unfinished agenda of infectious diseases and a rising, more challenging agenda of chronic diseases. The ongoing COVID-19 pandemic has stressed the health-care system like never before and laid bare all its flaws. India also has several opportunities in public health—it is an information and technology giant, the home of pharmaceutical and biotechnology industries, and has highly skilled clinicians, researchers and innovators—but they need to be deployed in the service of health.

The current Indian health-care system is a blend of public and private health-care providers, with various forms of medicine, including Western medicine (allopathy) and traditional medicines (Ayurveda, Siddha, Homoeopathy, Unani), largely co-existing. Despite a vast public health service infrastructure and a burgeoning private sector in health services, the populace is faced with challenges of poor accessibility and unaffordability, plus a treatment-based rather than a prevention-based model of health care. The lack of conceptual and operational interlinkages across the primary, secondary and tertiary levels of care contribute to the inadequate benefits of the available health services. Rural medical practitioners (RMPs), the first point of contact and highly trusted by the rural poor, fill some of the gaps. They provide affordable advice and counsel beyond health care, for example, helping the populace access medications and/or tests that may not be available in local pharmacies/laboratories. This informal network has helped many rural folks manage the challenge of getting health care and supply chain issues during the ongoing COVID-19 pandemic.

In this essay, we describe a new health-care paradigm that focuses on a continuum of quality care, from cradle to grave. We suggest that the focus of health-care needs to shift from vertical programmes looking at single diseases or conditions to a comprehensive, life-span approach, which begins from life in-utero, which will impact not only the health of the mother and child in the short term, but of the adult the child will grow into and the society at large (Fig. 1). These interventions need to address more than physical health and prioritize social determinants including nutrition, education, sanitation, habitation and respect for environment. We also introduce the concept of service integration across different facility levels (primary, secondary and tertiary care) for health services related to prevention, promotion, management, rehabilitation and palliation (Fig. 1).

The concept of continuity of care was embedded in the principles of Bhore Committee which was set up in 1943 to assess the health needs of the country and revitalized recently in the National Health Mission (NHM). The NHM envisages a health system where individuals can access equitable, affordable and quality health care across the lifespan (from conception to old age) for maternal and child health, adolescent health, communicable and non-communicable diseases at different facility levels. The

Figure 1: The New Health-Care Paradigm

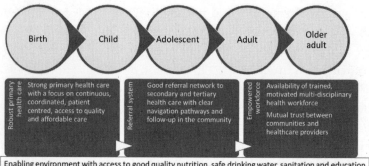

NHM was initially launched in rural India and then expanded to urban India. This is a three-tier system—primary health centres are the base, where frontline health workers, currently represented by the Accredited Social Health Activists (ASHAs) and multipurpose health workers link communities with doctors located at the centre. People may be referred from primary to secondary and tertiary care facilities, based on their health needs. In practice, however, many patients remain dependent on visits to specialists even for basic primary health care, with substantial delays, fragmentation of care and entirely avoidable health-care expenditure. The recently announced Health and Wellness Centres hold a lot of promise to improve access to quality and affordable preventive health care as articulated in the UN Sustainable Development Goals, but their success will depend on the transition from policy to implementation.

Let us take the example of chronic kidney disease, which is common, often coexists with other diseases, can progress from early to late stages of disease (with complications) and requires different interventions implemented at different levels of health care at all stages (Fig. 2) to illustrate how such integrated care can be delivered.

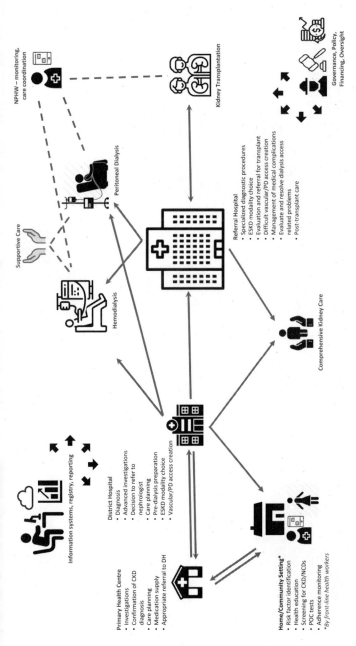

Primary Health Centre
- Investigations
- Confirmation of CKD diagnosis
- Care planning
- Medication supply
- Appropriate referral to DH

District Hospital
- Diagnosis
- Advanced investigations
- Decision to refer to nephrologist
- Care planning
- Pre-dialysis preparation
- ESKD modality choice
- Vascular/PD access creation

Home/Community Setting*
- Risk factor identification
- Health education
- Screening for CKD/NCDs
- POC tests
- Adherence monitoring
*By front-line health workers

Referral Hospital
- Specialized diagnostic procedures
- ESKD modality choice
- Evaluation and referral for transplant
- Difficult vascular/PD access creation
- Management of medical complications
- Evaluate and resolve dialysis access related problems
- Post-transplant care

Information systems, registry, reporting

NPHW – monitoring, care coordination

Supportive Care

Peritoneal Dialysis

Hemodialysis

Kidney Transplantation

Comprehensive Kidney Care

Governance, Policy, Financing, Oversight

Figure 2: How care could be delivered using a 'continuum of care' model for chronic kidney disease. Case finding takes place in the population and is conducted by frontline health-care workers. Essential preventative care and education is provided by a health-care worker with appropriate referral to primary care physician for care planning. Referral pathway is proposed in an escalating manner for care at secondary and tertiary levels according to disease severity. At all levels, the patient can return to the community for follow-up, monitoring and assessment of treatment adherence by the frontline health worker.

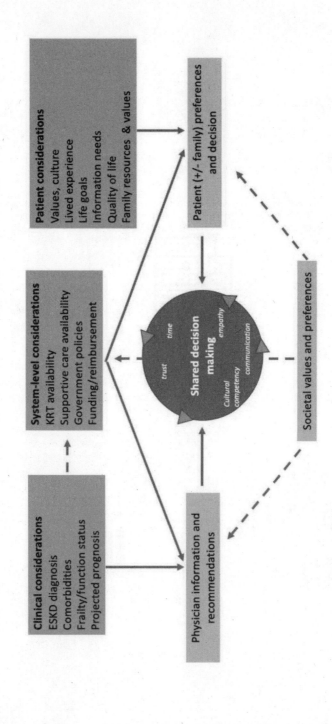

Areas of Health Care That Need Renewed Focus and Funding

Five areas of health care need renewed focus and energy: 1) safe motherhood and healthy childhood, 2) acute and chronic care, 3) conditions that can be eliminated, 4) chronic diseases and 5) mental health.

Securing a Healthy Start for Every Indian: Safe Motherhood, Healthy Childhood

Safe Motherhood: Gestational Diabetes Mellitus, Pregnancy-Induced Hypertension, Mental Health

India achieved the Millennium Development Goals (MDG) for maternal mortality—set at 139 deaths per 100,000 births—in 2016. This was due to a substantive increase in institutional deliveries, availability of skilled birth attendants, and programmes such as cash transfers to promote institutional deliveries. The momentum created by the MDGs and the National Health Mission (NHM) needs to be sustained with a focus on reducing the inequities between states. For example, in 2013, the maternal mortality rate for every 100,000 live births in Kerala was 61, while in Assam it was 300. For India to attain the goal of 70 deaths/10,00,000 live births by 2030, as listed in the sustainable development agenda, efforts need to continue towards bridging the rural–urban gap in health workforce and infrastructure needed to ensure consistent high-quality care during pregnancy, labour and delivery.

The large scale of under-nutrition in pregnant women is a significant challenge. Although micro and macro-nutrient deficiencies and infectious diseases are still a conundrum in reducing maternal morbidity, the presence of chronic diseases such as diabetes, hypertension, obesity and mental health conditions have created additional obstacles, thereby impacting safe motherhood and healthy childhood. According to the fourth National Family Health Survey, one in two pregnant women in India is anaemic. Pregnancy-induced hypertension and pre-eclampsia (a condition that involves many organs, including blood vessels, kidneys, liver and the haematological system, and has an adverse health impact on mother and baby) complicate between 8 and 10 per cent of all pregnancies. In addition, various surveys have shown that between two and twenty of all women develop diabetes during pregnancy (gestational diabetes mellitus), and 16–65 of every 100 women experience depression during and/or after delivery. The long-term physical or mental consequences resulting from these conditions during pregnancy and childbirth, referred to as postpartum morbidity, have a negative impact on the mother, newborn, family and the community. Women who develop high blood pressure or diabetes during pregnancy are at increased risk of developing diabetes, and heart and kidney diseases later in life, even if these conditions resolve immediately after delivery. Those with depression during pregnancy are at increased risk of chronic or recurrent depression, which impacts the growth and development of the baby as well as the health of the mother.

Unfortunately, the burden of these chronic diseases during pregnancy is not sufficiently recognized; they are not appropriately managed, and the long-term impacts not well understood. Maternity remains a neglected area of health care in India—poorly recognized, stigmatized and inadequately addressed. Innovative models of care are essential to address these chronic conditions which occur during an extremely important phase of life.

Child Health

Over the last seven decades, the Indian government has introduced several programmes aimed at improving child health.

The impact of these interventions is visible in the under-five mortality rate, which dramatically decreased from 126 per 1000 live births in 1990 to thirty-three per 1000 live births in 2020.[1] Although India missed achieving the MDG target for under-five mortality within the time frame, it achieved the goal a few years later. Besides being a measure of child health, under-five mortality is recognized as a superior measure of a health system because it reflects five years of potential intervention. The illnesses which cause under-five mortality are usually preventable, treatable or both, and most common in low-income settings. One of the best, most unbiased methods to understand the effect of a country's health-care policies on its populace, therefore, is to look at under-five mortality.

Even though immunization is universally available across all public health centres in India, in 2016, 63 per cent of children aged 12–23 months received full vaccination (three doses of diphtheria-pertussis and tetanus vaccine, one of Bacillus-Calmette-Guerin, one dose of measles, mumps and rubella vaccine).[2] India ranks second (after Nigeria) in the number of children unvaccinated against measles and performs the worst amongst all developing countries, with 35 per cent of children being underweight and 38 per cent stunted. It is estimated that 16–18 per cent of babies born in India are low birth weight (<2.5 kg).[3, 4, 5] Low birth weight has a long-term impact on chronic diseases later in life; these children are susceptible to risk factors such as diabetes, insulin susceptibility and hypertension, leading to chronic diseases such as diabetes, kidney disease and heart disease. In stark contrast, over-nutrition and obesity are becoming increasingly common among older children and adolescents, leading to the early onset of conditions such as high blood pressure and diabetes. These societal and economic changes warrant the need for policies and programmes which are comprehensive, integrated and adopt a life-course approach to health, physical activity and nutrition.

Impact of Gender-Based Norms on Access to Health Care

Biologically, women live longer than men, but have fewer years of quality health care. Alongside low socioeconomic status, skewed gender norms and low education levels are likely critical determinants of social exclusion and consequent ill-health. Due to entrenched patriarchal norms in India, women's health needs tend not to be prioritized, particularly when there are costs associated with care. This is primarily due to traditional norms wherein most women are treated as second-class citizens—responsible for unpaid and household duties, and not involved in decision-making—and hence have restricted access to social benefits, including health care. India has one of the world's worst sex ratios, with an excess of thirty-seven million males. According to the 2011 census, there is a 17 per cent gap in literacy between males and females. Even when girls are enrolled in school, they are more likely to drop out. Furthermore, women are subjected to violence and discrimination. In 2016, the National Family Health Survey found that one in three women have been subjected to domestic violence. The National Crime Report Bureau reported that three dowry deaths took place each day in 2017, and in 2019, the Crimes in India Report registered eighty-seven rape cases every day. Discrimination against the girl child and gender-based violence violate basic human rights, have a long-term impact on the health and wellness of the survivor's life, and need to be confronted using a whole-of-society approach. Alongside a poorly coordinated, under-resourced and fragmented health system, these cultural challenges result in a substantial number of women suffering from the consequences of ill-health and dying before reaching a treatment facility. Women also suffer the adverse health consequences of entirely preventable conditions, like cervical cancer.

Navigating this challenge requires the development of comprehensive and integrated services, and a woman-centred model of care which begins with educating adolescent girls and women, bringing them into the workforce and making available screening, diagnosis, referral, management and follow-up for risk factors or diseases in the community. The introduction of ASHAs, resident female community health workers, has created opportunities to empower women in rural India, where ASHAs are often seen as role models who care for mothers and children and speak up for women's rights. Another success story comes from the self-help group movement, which has 67 million members across India. These groups empower women through entrepreneurial training, livelihood promotion activities, financial and social support, and addressing a range of issues including domestic violence, caste-related issues and financial stability that are likely to increase their involvement in their own and their family members' health.

Addressing the Need for Acute and Chronic Care: Early and Sustained Response

Acute care is a continuum in patient care, starting from triage, early management, transport to the nearest hospital, including to the emergency room and intensive care facilities when needed, and post-discharge follow-up. It is relevant across a range of conditions from injuries such as road traffic crashes and snakebites, acute presentations of chronic conditions such as heart attack and stroke, infectious diseases such as diarrhoea and emerging conditions like COVID-19.

India accounts for 10 per cent of global road traffic crashes while it has only 1 per cent of the world's vehicles.[6] Recognizing this, the Government of India is developing a network of trauma care centres across the country. The 108-emergency toll-free number under a public-private partnership was launched in 2005 in Andhra Pradesh to improve emergency response services (primarily ambulances) and has now been implemented across thirty-one states and union territories. The government's plans include establishing an emergency medical care centre and a trauma care centre for every district, along with ambulance and paramedical personnel so that no trauma victim needs to be transported more than 50 km to a designated hospital. These emergency centres would potentially manage a range of acute illnesses and prevent premature mortality.

Critical care, a discipline of medicine which cares for people with life-threatening conditions, requires an intensive care unit with machines to monitor vital signs and provide life-support and a team of specially trained health-care providers. It garnered global attention during the current pandemic, in particular the second surge in 2021. In 2020, India had only 2.3 intensive care unit beds per 100,000 population (compared to 12.9 beds per 100,000 population in Canada), and relatively few doctors and allied health personnel (nurses, technicians) with intensive care training.[7] Nevertheless, critical care is evolving rapidly in urban India in terms of training opportunities, availability of intensive care beds and state-of-the-art equipment. The pandemic has underscored the need to be prepared to ensure adequate delivery of intensive care to critically ill patients.

The third type of acute care is care for acute presentation of chronic diseases such as heart attack and stroke. The goal of this type of care is speedy assessment and management of patients to increase their chance of surviving the condition, maximizing their recovery and reducing their risk of another incident. These conditions require (i) early recognition of symptoms, (ii) urgent testing to determine the cause and guide treatment, (iii) facilities to initiate treatments (such as aspirin and thrombolytic therapy) or procedures (angioplasty), (iv) multidisciplinary team-based care, (v) secondary prevention and (vi) rehabilitation. The capacity to provide these services has improved rapidly in urban India over the last twenty-five years. For rural India, unfortunately, this remains a distant dream—while referral pathways have been established, most referral centres lack basic infrastructure and human resources to initiate and continue treatment for these conditions. Loss of precious time leads to a large number of avoidable deaths. According to the Management of Acute Coronary Event Registry of the Indian Council of Medical Research, every other heart attack victim in India takes more than six and a half hours to reach a hospital, which is almost thirteen times more than the ideal window of thirty minutes.[8]

For those fortunate to survive such an event, continuity of care during the transition from acute to chronic care is essential and is a core component of high-performing health-care systems.

Disease Conditions That Can Be Eliminated: Ambitions and Strategies

Eradication (permanent global reduction to zero of a disease) or elimination (reduction of a disease to zero from a region or country) of disease is the goal of public health. Usually, the World Health Organization sets the goal for eradication and countries work towards achieving elimination. The world has cooperated and worked hard to eliminate two diseases to date: smallpox and rinderpest. Smallpox, caused by variola virus, was a debilitating, highly contagious disease that killed 300 million people in the twentieth century alone. The control of smallpox came about by a vaccination created by Edward Jenner in 1796. It took almost two centuries from the creation of the vaccine to the declaration of eradication on 8 May 1980.

Diseases that can potentially be eradicated need to fulfil some basic criteria—they need to be easily diagnosable, infect only humans (presence in non-human vectors allows reinfection and spread) and be geographically restricted. With rare exceptions, disease eradication requires availability of an effective vaccine.

Some of the vaccine-preventable conditions that can be eliminated include the following, with effective vaccines already available for the first three conditions:

1. Poliomyelitis (caused by polio virus): India, which had 60 per cent of global polio cases till 2009, was able to rid itself of polio through concerted action. India had its last case of polio in 2011 and was officially declared polio-free in 2014. In August 2020, Africa was declared free of wild polio.
2. Measles and rubella: Measles and rubella have been eliminated in the Americas, European and Western Pacific Region. India needs to achieve and maintain population immunity by providing high vaccination coverage of measles and rubella vaccines.
3. Cervical cancer: Caused by human papilloma virus (HPV), cervical cancer is preventable. For successful elimination, all countries must reach and maintain an annual incidence rate of below four per 1,00,000 women. The global strategy for elimination includes vaccinating over 90 per cent of girls by the age of fifteen, screening of more than 70 per cent of women by thirty-five years of age and management of invasive cancer cases.
4. Rheumatic heart disease caused by Streptococcus A bacteria. A vaccine will likely be required for its prevention.

The Chronic Disease Burden and Its Management: Realities and Mitigation Strategies

In addition to infectious and undernutrition-related illnesses, India has been experiencing a rising burden of chronic non-infectious or non-communicable diseases (NCD) and injuries such as road traffic crash, drowning and violence over the last thirty years. In 2016, more than 61 per cent of all deaths were due to chronic diseases.[9] State-wise analyses of disease burden show that more people now die of chronic disease and injuries than infectious and maternal and child health-related conditions in all states.[10] This transition from communicable diseases to NCDs as the major cause of death happened at different times in different states, with Kerala and Goa the first two to make this transition.

Compared to Western countries, chronic diseases in the Indians develop at a younger age, are associated with unique and poorly studied risk factors and impact the economically productive section of society. For example, Indians develop adverse consequences of obesity at a lower body mass index compared to the Western population. This is postulated to be due to disproportionately increased distribution of body fat around the abdomen (e.g. central obesity). There are likely unique risk factors, possibly getting exacerbated by new health challenges like environment change. For example, the incidence of kidney disease without any known risk factor (such as diabetes or hypertension) developing in young people engaged in agricultural activities in hot and humid environments.[11]

Chronic diseases such as stroke, cancer and kidney disease require lifelong care. Such care is largely delivered in disease-specific silos by specialists, usually in private sector hospitals, located away from rural areas. Significant concerns have been raised with regard to private sector health care, which has a focus on profit and is alleged to engage in excessive and often unnecessary testing, use unproven and unnecessary therapies, and harbour misaligned incentives because of the involvement of the pharmaceutical industry.

Unlike acute illnesses, these diseases do not produce symptoms in early stages, hence affected individuals do not seek medical care. This leads to loss of crucial opportunities to intervene and prevent development of complications. Further, long-term chronic disease management leads to enormous out-of-pocket payments, and people often have to make the difficult choice of suffering the consequences of no treatment, or to push their families into poverty due to the treatment expenses. Especially challenging is the acute presentation of chronic diseases, which typically requires expensive, technology-intensive care. People find themselves in a position where they are presented with a limited set of choices and are asked to decide without having access to full information. Finally, chronic diseases also develop in clusters, a condition called multi-morbidity, which makes it imperative that health system response be coordinated rather than develop in disease-specific silos.

Given these challenges, the country needs a multipronged approach to management, starting from upstream, broad-based interventions that force a change in the default choices to healthier ones—for example, imposition of tax on tobacco and alcohol, promoting the availability and consumption of locally sourced fruits and vegetables through existing platforms like the public distribution system or inclusion in mid-day meals, development of more pedestrian- and cycling-friendly road and transport systems, improving health education and promotion and, importantly, shifting the dial from cure to prevention through evidence-based guidelines, accessible, community-based multi-disciplinary teams supported by low-cost technology. With a focus on quality improvement, primary health care should become the first contact of the population with the health system, and care should be continuous, comprehensive, coordinated and people-centred, responsive to the values and preferences of the society. Setting up health and wellness centres, introduction of mid-level health providers and up-skilling of multipurpose workers and ASHAs to promote prevention and control of chronic diseases are promising and will bring about a new era focusing on low-cost prevention and promotion that will build trust in the system, rather than hospital-based, expensive curative health care (Figure 1).

Mental Wellbeing

According to the Global Burden of Disease Study, in 2017, one out of seven Indians was affected by mental disorders such as depression and anxiety. The National Mental Health Survey 2016 suggested that approximately 150 million Indians needed active interventions for mental health conditions. The gap between those who needed and received treatment ranged from 70–92 per cent for different disorders. The total number of years lost to illness, disability or premature death attributed to mental, neurological and substance-use disorders in India increased by 61 per cent between 1990 and 2013, and is estimated to show a further 23 per cent increase by 2025. India spends just 1.3 per cent of its health budget on mental health, much less than other nations. This translates into productivity-linked economic losses—India is projected to lose $1.03 trillion before 2030 due to mental health conditions.[12]

These sobering data call for a rights-based approach to mental health that uses tailored, evidence-based, easily accessible interventions that cover both clinical and social aspects of these conditions. Although several policy reforms have been made, including the introduction of a National Mental Health Programme and a Mental Healthcare Act, these are poorly implemented and inadequately accessed. India needs an integrated approach to educate the public, screen, diagnose, treat and manage patients with mental health conditions. Low-cost, high-quality, evidence-based interventions using the available health workforce have been developed and led by Indian researchers but are yet to be scaled up and decentralized. Equally important is to start normalizing the discourse on mental health and raising awareness about the condition. Families, communities, school and the media need to play a part in reducing stigma and discrimination associated with mental health.

Patient-Centred Care as a Catalyst for Change

Involvement of the public in health care—both in the delivery of care and generation of new knowledge through research—has emerged as central towards creating a climate of trust where patients and health-care professionals can integrate modern medicine with traditional care, cultural beliefs, social values and preferences in the overall context of collective memory. Individuals and families should be able to share their lived experiences with health-care providers that so that the issues that matter to patients can be prioritized. This process of full information sharing and assessment of available options allows shared and tailored decision-making, whether in the hospital, clinic or community. From a passive recipient of instructions, the patient becomes a member of the care team while the health-care provider become a patient advocate and strives to provide safe and effective care. Such care paradigms have been shown to lead to higher rates of patient satisfaction, adherence to suggested lifestyle changes and prescribed treatment, continuity during transition, better outcomes and more cost-effective care.

Public Trust in the Health-Care System

Finally, the role of public trust is key in the health-care system. As the experience to contain the COVID-19 outbreak, centered around an effective vaccine against SARS-CoV2, has highlighted, disease elimination requires sustained political, financial, social, global and individual efforts. Public trust is central to this process. In recent times, a concerning development is the fear and mistrust in science, and reliance on conspiracy theories—as seen by the rise in anti-vaccination movement. Easy access of information online and the use of social media and fake news has altered the dynamics of patient–doctor communications and blurred the boundaries between science and fiction. In order to overcome these headwinds, the scientific world needs to be able to communicate clearly, effectively and build trust between patients and health professionals. The US government's national strategy for the COVID-19 response and pandemic preparedness identified 'Restoring trust with the American people' as goal number 1. In his letter to the citizens immediately after assuming office, President Joe Biden committed to be 'honest and transparent . . . about both the good news and the bad'. Policies and legislations need to be clear, consistent with societal values and preferences and transparently applied. Policymakers should incentivize measures backed by science and be prepared to look beyond short-term partisan gains to achieve long-term goals.

India's health care is in urgent need of relationship building between the health system, the provider and the patient. Trust, which is the foundation of this relationship, results from the patient's judgement of the doctor's technical and communication skills, the patient's perception of how the system works as well as the reputation of the doctor and/or the hospital. Trust is critical to mitigate the vulnerability, uncertainty and unpredictability inherent to the provision of health care, and depends on the availability of a competent health workforce, the perception that the system acts in the best interest of the patient and honest communication between the patient and the doctor.

Trust in the health system is at an all-time low in India, as evident in the recent increase in violence against doctors, even before the COVID-19 pandemic; as illness is accompanied by feelings of vulnerability, changes in position of power, and uncertainty about the future, it is critical that people are able to believe that they will get consistent and good quality care. The genesis of the loss of trust is multifactorial, ultimately based on the assumption of lack of benevolent agency or altruistic motives on the part of those providing health care and poor communication. Social media creates an echo chamber that reinforces such beliefs. Lack of trust manifests in many forms, many detrimental to patient's health—such as doubting doctors' motives leading to failure to follow medical advice and getting drawn to unproven, 'miracle' cures. The ever-worsening state of public hospitals due to chronic shortage of doctors and other staff, medical equipment, drugs and space, forces the population to seek care in the private sector even when it is unaffordable. The high cost of care combined with shared experiences of commercialization and managerialism, manifested in overbilling and unnecessary prescriptions, procedures and diagnostics, create a vicious cycle of mistrust and resentment. With easy access to technology, people are seeking information from the internet and social media, which has impacted their trust and confidence in health-care providers.

Better communication and compassion, integrity and ethics in clinical care, focusing on patient satisfaction and building a rapport with patients will eventually translate to improving trust between the patient and provider. Another method of improving this trust is by involving community members in planning and monitoring health services and keeping the system, including patients, doctors and the hospital management, accountable.

Health is a fundamental human right, and access to affordable health care is an important priority for governments.

The Supreme Court of India has held that the fundamental right to live with human dignity, enshrined in Article 21, includes protection of health. Hence access to affordable health care should be an important priority for governments. As Indians face acute and chronic illnesses, newly emerging infections and injuries, the health system needs to be responsive to these demands. The COVID-19 pandemic has exposed the structural flaws in India's health-care system. The silver lining, however, is the mainstreaming of conversation on health care and the realization of the need to build a resilient, responsive, trustworthy and sustainable system. All stakeholders need to pull in the same direction to ensure that services are delivered in an efficient, trustworthy and cost-effective way. Whether India can develop a health-care system that is accessible, affordable, provides quality patient-centred health care by a motivated and trained multidisciplinary team, is comprehensive and continuous in providing prevention, cure and palliation, without any discrimination and inequity to its citizens is still in the realms of uncertainty. The health sector alone cannot bring about these changes and needs to work in partnership with the education sector, social services, water and sanitation and infrastructure. The time is now: India needs to invest and start transforming this vision into reality.

Building Equitable and Responsive Hospitals: Lessons from the Indian Experience

Ramani Atkuri and Pavitra Mohan

'How do we draw the lessons learnt from a pre-COVID world to the present day? The challenges are many: the health situation has worsened; people are more impoverished; the social determinants of health are badly affected; people's ability to access care, as well as all levels of care from primary to tertiary have been badly affected. In such a scenario how do we ensure universal health care?'

—Dr Anand Zachariah, professor of medicine,
Christian Medical College, Vellore

Introduction

The COVID-19 pandemic exposed the poor state of public hospitals in India. Inadequate infrastructure—from beds, oxygen, ventilators and drugs to staff—led to thousands of deaths. Years of underinvestment in public health and a simultaneous expansion of private hospitals with a nominal public–private partnership (PPP) has resulted in a near-defunct system of secondary and tertiary health care. The so-called PPP has only meant that prime land has been leased out at nominal costs, amenities are provided on easy terms and charges, and quality of care is unchecked. However, as we will proceed to show in this essay, it is possible to not only provide good quality secondary and tertiary care to patients, but to provide it at a reasonable cost.

The 75th NSSO Report (2017–18) on health in India found that the utilization of public hospitals for inpatient care had remained largely the same in rural areas over the past twenty-five years—from 44 per cent in 1995–96 to 46 per cent in 2017–18. In urban areas, on the other hand, the use of public hospitals for in-patient care declined; it fell from 43 per cent to 38 per cent in the same time period. Utilization of NGO-run or trust hospitals was low too and stayed at around 2–4 per cent of all hospitalizations.[1] While most (90 per cent) admissions in government hospitals were free, 25 per cent patients received free care in NGO-run/trust hospitals, and only about 3 per cent received free care in private hospitals.

Between August and September 2020, we studied four secondary and two tertiary hospitals in the non-governmental sector, with the aim of sieving out lessons for public and private hospitals to provide responsive and high-quality care at affordable costs. Four of these hospitals are located in tribal areas: Tribal Health Initiative Hospital (THI) at Sittilingi in Tamil Nadu; Christian Hospital at Bissam Cuttack in Odisha (CHB); Jan Swasthya Sahyog (JSS) at Ganiyari in Chhattisgarh and Shaheed Hospital (SH) at Dalli Rajhara in Chhattisgarh. Two are tertiary care hospitals: Cachar Cancer Hospital and Research Centre (CCH) at Silchar, Assam and the Christian Medical College and Hospital (CMCH) at Vellore, Tamil Nadu.[2]

How do these non-profit hospitals manage to function at a fraction of the cost of private health-care providers? How do they maintain good quality at a lower cost? Is it possible to leverage their availability and experiences for strengthening public hospitals and guiding the private ones? How can their design and principles be leveraged to enable provision of universal health care to all Indians, of a quality they deserve and at a cost they can afford? These are some of the questions we explore in this paper.

What Makes Non-profit Organizations Effective Health-Care Providers?

We examined the non-profit hospitals in our study in terms of the following characteristics: organization of services; management structures; financing; community-based programmes; linkages with government and other non-governmental organizations, and their role in informing health policies and programmes.

Organization of Services

All the hospitals we studied were acutely conscious of how expensive and indebting it can be for a family to seek health care. These non-profit hospitals were driven by the vision of providing high-quality, affordable health care to people in need. For example, the Cachar Cancer Hospital vision explicitly states: 'no patient is denied appropriate cancer treatment for want of resources.' Similarly, Aravind Eye Hospital's vision is to provide compassionate and quality eye care to all. This is the mission statement of JSS, Ganiyari: '. . . developing a low-cost and effective health programme that provides both preventive and curative services in the tribal and rural areas of Bilaspur and surrounding areas of Chhattisgarh in central India. We strongly believe that access to health care should not be denied to anyone due to lack of money or due to discrimination on account of caste, sex, religion and social class etc.'

These hospitals are determined not to let their health care impoverish families or to deny anyone access for lack of money.

Their focus on equity, affordability and non-discrimination based on ability to pay is noteworthy. Most of these hospitals started where there were no other services available and where marginalized populations live. JSS is located, for instance, outside Bilaspur and serves the landless scheduled-caste and scheduled-tribe agricultural labourers living in the forest villages of Achanakmar sanctuary. CHB works in western Odisha, which is known for its high poverty levels, and is situated 50 km from the district headquarters.

Availability and Accessibility

Located in rural areas or in small towns, these hospitals are more accessible than those located in block or district headquarters. The Cachar Cancer Hospital in Silchar, for instance, is 350 km from Guwahati where the other cancer hospital is located, a journey that can take up to twenty hours by road. Some hospitals are constructed in the local design with locally available materials, making the institution a familiar and non-threatening place for the local population (Figure 1).

Having local staff in the hospital who can speak the region's language or dialect goes a long way in helping patients negotiate their way in the hospital and making it feel less alien. In the THI hospital at Sittilingi, apart from the three doctors and a nurse, all the other staff (including nurses, lab technicians and radiologists) are tribal men and women, recruited locally and then trained in the required specialty.

Further, health services are available round the clock—a very important aspect of accessibility. Apart from maternity services, emergency care is available day and night. Stocking of essential emergency drugs like oxygen, as well as of anti-snake venom and anti-rabies vaccine by these hospitals has saved many lives over the years. Non-availability of these drugs in the peripheral public health system, and inability of patients to purchase these from the market costs many a life.

Figure 1: The Original OPD block of Jan Swasthya Sahyog, Ganiyari

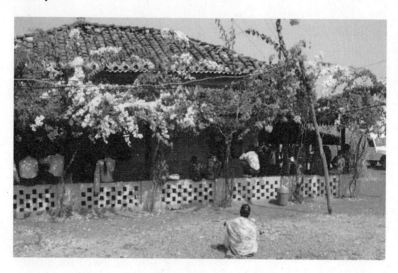

One of the common threads running through these health-care institutions is the attitude of the staff towards patients and their relatives. Polite and empathetic, they make the patients feel valued as people at a time when they are already scared and worried about their or their family member's illness. Senior staff in the hospital actively work to develop a team spirit among all the staff members, of working towards a common purpose of service and empathetic care. Staff learn and are motivated by observing how senior management behave with patients and their relatives.

Affordability

An active effort is made to keep the costs as low as possible. Everyone is conscious of the opportunity costs of seeking care, hence consultation, investigations, diagnosis and management plan are all sought to be completed in a single day. This reduces the days of wages lost for the patient and her attendants.

Consultation fees ranged from Rs 10–20 and inpatient charges from Rs 10–30 per day. Drugs and investigations are charged so as to recover their costs, with a maximum additional margin of 10 per cent. Drugs used are largely generics, procured from organizations like LOCOST (Low-Cost Standard Therapeutics, Vadodara) or CDMU (Community Development Medicinal Unit), apart from some local procurement, which reduces costs. Inpatient costs are also kept low by having functional but not luxurious wards.

Opportunity costs are reduced by providing accommodation to the patients and attendants in a *dharamshala*. While the dharamshala is necessary for relatives of inpatients, many outpatients too need this facility due to poor public transport facilities in these regions, necessitating an overnight stay before the patient can return home the next day by the next available transport. Jan Swasthya Sahyog and the Shaheed Hospital at Dalli Rajhara also provided stoves for patients to cook their own meals while staying in the dharamshala. It is not unusual to see patients come to the clinic accompanied by one or two attendants bringing with them cooking utensils, firewood and some rice, pulses and potatoes.

These hospitals also run an ambulance service to bring emergency cases to the hospital when required. States like Chhattisgarh and Odisha have no public transport system and, often, the government-run ambulance services do not reach remote rural or tribal areas, or take too long to reach. In such situations, provision of ambulance services can save lives and money.

Use of Rational Therapy Regimens and Appropriate Technology

There is an unwavering commitment to keep treatment rational, minimize investigations, medication and hospital stay—crucial to keeping costs to the patient low and optimizing health effects. Only the most essential investigations are ordered and diagnostic algorithms and standard treatment protocols are used to ensure accuracy of diagnosis and rationality of treatment.

Innovations such as a low-cost electrophoresis machine for diagnosis of sickle cell disease; breath counters to aid diagnosis of childhood pneumonia and an easy-to-read thermometer for diagnosing fever by community health workers, among others, help to reduce costs, as well as improve access to health care at the periphery and at the facility. Purification of water with the use of ultraviolet light is another instance of putting appropriate, low-cost technology to use. Using mosquito nets for the repair of hernias, as is done in THI, Sittilingi, is yet another instance.

Quality of Care

Highest quality of care, regardless of ability to pay, is the central philosophy driving these hospitals. Having a well-functioning laboratory is thus an essential component of such institutions. A laboratory conducting basic microbiological, hematological and biochemical tests keeps costs low by helping to make correct diagnoses and deciding appropriate treatment without wasting resources. Since many tests are now automated, it is easier for small hospitals to conduct these tests.

Basic specialties of general medicine, pediatrics, obstetrics and general surgery are provided at all hospitals, with most doctors becoming multi-skilled *rural generalists* and managing all types of patients. At JSS, Ganiyari, surgical expertise extends to even major surgeries like cancer surgery and reconstructive surgery, which is generally considered tertiary level of care.

Other specialties like psychiatry, dental care, eye care and cardiology are managed by periodic visits by external consultants, who come on a fixed day to see patients. Tie-ups with nearby specialty care hospitals has facilitated procedures like dialysis or cardiac surgery, often at a concessional price.

Equity

Most NGO-run hospitals do not make any distinction between rich and poor patients and do not have private rooms. When they do, they use the higher charges in private rooms to cross-subsidize poorer patients. For example, in Christian Hospital, Bissam Cuttack, when patients choose a private room for inpatient care, all charges such as investigations and bed charges are higher. Some hospitals charge their 'target audience', such as tribals, less than they charge others. However, others (like Cachar Cancer Hospital) do not have differential charges, believing that once some patients pay more for services and others do not, these 'private' patients start demanding more attention and sooner or later, the focus of the hospital shifts to them at the cost of poorer patients.

Another feature often found is that of a facilitator who guides and even accompanies patients if they need to access a service in a large hospital. For instance, it is almost impossible for a tribal from a village in Chhattisgarh to negotiate their way to the medical college in Raipur to find out where they can get their Anti-Retroviral Therapy for HIV infection or radiation therapy for cancer. Just having someone accompany them on this journey makes access to care more equitable.

Social Determinants of Health

Almost all the hospitals addressed some social determinant of health. JSS, for example, addresses the problem of childhood malnutrition through the setting up of crèches in the community for young children. Since the nutritional status of a patient directly affects the health outcome, the hospital provides a protein- and calorie-rich diet to all inpatients, as well as a nutrient-rich mix for debilitated patients. THI encourages economic activity in the villages around the hospital through organic farming, promotion of local craft and setting up farmers' cooperatives, all of which have served to improve the economic status of the community. Christian Hospital, Bissam Cuttack, had started a school for tribal children, with teachers from the tribal community, as a means of empowerment.

Financing

Though inpatients are charged nominally (around Rs 30 per day), surgeries are often charged higher. Income from surgical procedures often subsidizes other care. Social insurance schemes also help in subsidizing costs, even though only a section of the patients are covered by them. Usually, migrants and those who live deep in the forests are uninsured. The Rashtriya Swasthya Bima Yojana (RSBY) paid for inpatient treatment for some patients earlier, but has now been replaced by the Pradhan Mantri Jan Arogya Yojana (PMJAY) under the Ayushman Bharat (AB) programme. In two of the hospitals studied (Jan Swasthya Sahyog, Ganiyari and Shaheed Hospital, Dalli Rajhara), a significant number of inpatients were enrolled in the AB scheme. Since the rates fixed by the government are higher than the charges usually levied by the non-profit hospitals, the scheme's reimbursement provides extra funds to further subsidize those not enrolled in AB. However, there have been difficulties in getting expenses reimbursed, especially beyond the first Rs 50,000.

Apart from patient charges and reimbursement from PMJAY, some non-profits obtain grants—either from funding agencies such as Tata Trusts or from the government—to cover partial costs. Some of them get individual donations as well towards their work.

Several organizations reported that they are now independent of external funding as patient collections are enough for salaries, drugs and consumables, as well as for maintenance of buildings and equipment. The collections also enable them to provide free treatment for those who cannot afford care. This is even without patients availing the government insurance schemes. The hospitals often require funding only for capital expansion. However, in extremely poor regions (as in many parts of India), it is not possible for patients to pay for their health care, unless subsidized either by the government as in public hospitals, through insurance, cross-subsidizing or by external funding. In such instances, charging even low fees for services runs the risk of keeping away the very poor.

At Cachar Cancer Hospital, diagnosis is made within two days and a treatment plan prepared. Caregivers who cannot afford to lose wages are given ad hoc employment on campus—in the garden or kitchen or as assistant to the electrician or plumber. They are provided food and a daily wage of Rs 250. Patients pay a one-time lifetime registration charge for cancer care and for lifelong dental care. Since patients do not have to keep paying, compliance with treatment has increased. Costs for cancer care are reimbursed from the PMJAY or the state-funded health insurance for those who cannot pay. A third of CMCH's patients are private patients who pay more than the cost price of services, a third are subsidized, and another third are treated free of cost. The high patient turnover allows them to be self-sufficient.

Costs to the patients are also directly linked to the salary paid to the staff in the hospital, most significantly to the doctors. In all the non-profit hospitals that we studied, the medical, paramedical and other staff are paid much less than their counterparts in the public or private sectors. By keeping salaries low, the overall costs of running the service are also brought down. However, a stimulating work environment, learning opportunities and a sense of community and purpose keeps the team motivated. Availability of accommodation within the campus helps staff stay with their families comfortably. CH, Bissam Cuttack, also runs an English-medium school in the town, which provides a good standard of education to children of the town and of the hospital staff.

Outreach and Community-Based Initiatives

Most of the secondary hospitals that we studied provide outreach services and engage in community-based initiatives. Outreach clinics help to provide early care, detect more serious cases to refer them to the hospital and provide continuity of care through follow up of discharged patients.

Community health workers or nurses improve the impact of services. For example, purely hospital-based treatment of tuberculosis results in poorer compliance than when a patient diagnosed with tuberculosis is checked up on by the community health worker or nurse. Screening for serious illnesses can be done and illnesses like malaria can be diagnosed early. Pregnant women with risk factors can be detected and referred. A patient treated and discharged from the hospital has access to follow-up care in the village through them.

Even tertiary hospitals such as Christian Medical College and Hospital (CMCH) stress the need to keep links with the community as it improves trust and faith in the hospital. CMCH runs community programmes (Community Health and Development unit and the Rural Unit for Health and Social Affairs), and cases not requiring tertiary care are managed there. Community activities include preventive activities like screening for non-communicable diseases and health education.

The Cachar Cancer Hospital provides chemotherapy and palliative care through outreach clinics. Two satellite centres see patients from the two adjacent districts in the Barak valley. The team here believes that many aspects of cancer care—prevention, palliative care, rehabilitation—are dependent on the community more than on the facilities and, therefore, community engagement and involvement is key.

Management of the Hospital and Staff

When hospitals initially came up in remote, rural and backward areas (like the one in Sittilingi, for instance), they began by training local staff (who may or may not have completed high school) in the basics of nursing. Over time, these women and men become knowledgeable and skilled at nursing care. However, they are not recognized by the government as they are not formally trained. Hence, the NGOs have had to either ensure their nurses received formal training, or had to recruit qualified nurses to comply with the Clinical Establishment Act, even though their knowledge and skill may be poorer than the ones trained in-house. Most other staff—radiographers, lab technicians—are locally recruited and trained or sent for training as required. Doctors are also sent for further training depending on the services required by the hospital, such as pediatrics, obstetrics, anaesthesiology, surgery.

Most of the hospitals we studied are registered as Trusts or Societies and have a General Body and Executive Committee or a Management Committee. The management participates in the day-to-day working of the hospital, with representatives from different hospital services being part of the working committee or a steering committee. Nurses are given a larger role in management and decision-making than is seen in public hospitals.

Feedback about how the hospital is functioning is obtained variously from health workers in the community (JSS); from famers' collectives and local staff (THI); and from patient feedback forms (CMCH). All policies or policy changes made by the Cachar Cancer Centre's policies have to be ratified by the Cachar Cancer Society, which is made up of local community members only, with no representatives of the hospital.

Linkages with Government and with Other Institutions

While the hospitals studied are recognized by the government for services such as safe deliveries (women delivering here receive JSY money) or TB care (some are DOTS centres), there is a level of wariness between the health authorities and the NGOs. Involvement in local government programmes depends on the respective health officers at a given point of time. While one officer in charge may seek inputs and help from the NGOs, others may view them with suspicion.

CMCH has initiated a distance-learning programme on family medicine for government doctors. It also runs distance courses in psychiatry, geriatrics and diabetes. So, instead of trying to get urban doctors to move to rural areas, they focus on doctors already located in rural areas and empower them with better knowledge and skills. This programme is being availed of by different state governments as well for their physicians posted in the periphery. The hospital also has links with other peripheral mission hospitals round the country, and there is a regular exchange of consultants from CMCH to the periphery to fill short vacancies, or to teach; while the peripheral doctors come to the teaching hospital when they need in-house training. Keeping links with the community also enables the teaching hospital to be in touch with realities at ground level.

Some organizations train and build capacity of health workers and the professional staff of other NGO-run health facilities. However, as these hospitals grow, their doctors and nurses find less time for training staff of other organizations, which is a pity. Capacity building of smaller and newer organizations is a significant contribution many of these hospitals could make. Creation of networks of similar secondary-care hospitals will enable them to better play the role of advocates for rational, low-cost, high-quality care, apart from mutual support and learning.

At present, nine secondary-care hospitals have come together to support a rural fellowship for young medical professionals, to enable them to work for a year or more to understand the reality of rural India. Each fellow doctor spends four months each in three of the nine institutions. They have a mentor who guides them through the year, as well as a local mentor in each organization that the fellow spends their time in. It is hoped that such an exposure will enthuse some of them to take up work in small rural hospitals in future. Christian Medical College, Vellore, networks with several secondary-care hospitals in rural areas where medical students are sent during their third and fourth year for a period of two to three weeks, as an exposure to working with limited resources. They get to see the vast difference in conditions of work in rural and even remote areas when compared to a tertiary teaching hospital, though rural hospitals too get very complex cases to manage.

In many cases, these hospitals have established linkages with private providers or hospitals where they refer patients for more advanced care. Usually, they negotiate lower rates than what the hospital charges. When specialists are called to the hospital for procedures, or for consultation, the fees paid is less than what the specialist would normally charge in a city hospital.

Role in Advocacy

Its close ties to the community and careful documentation of disease patterns as well as trends in nutritional status have enabled JSS to advocate for and influence policy changes in different areas. Similarly, Christian Hospital has helped inform and support the malaria-malnutrition programme in Odisha. Tertiary institutions like CMCH, too, use research conducted in the hospital and in the field for policy advocacy purposes. CMCH was instrumental in shaping the national policy for leprosy management and, more recently, for the management of HIV/AIDS. Rotavirus vaccine research was also carried out in CMCH.

Conclusions and Lessons

Admittedly, we have taken a small sample of the hospitals for the study; there are many more that deliver high-quality and ethical care to the underserved populations, at a cost they can afford. Though the sampled hospitals are located in rural / tribal areas or in smaller towns, we believe hospitals located anywhere in India can draw valuable lessons from how they function.

Secondary hospitals run by NGOs / non-profit organizations show several ways to deliver better health care. Their focus on keeping costs low and conserving resources is something that can and should be taken up by all other hospitals. This goes hand in hand with ensuring adequate facilities supporting clinical care at the hospital—whether it is a laboratory with the requisite reagents and an appropriately trained lab technician, or a pharmacy with a well-functioning inventory control system and no stock-outs. Such measures save the patient time and cost in getting tests done outside or procuring branded medicines from the market.

An empathetic and caring environment puts patients at ease and creates trust, also allowing hospitals to understand the users' needs and address them, for instance, by providing for basic conveniences for patients' and their attendants' stay. Having services available round the clock, including that of a physician, is essential. To that extent, proper accommodation on the campus of the block CHC for essential staff is necessary.

These hospitals illustrate the urgent need for government-run secondary care hospitals (CHCs and district hospitals) to build stronger linkages with the community through the health sub-centres (SCs) and the primary health centres (PHCs). Back referrals to PHCs and SCs from CHCs and DHs will reduce the rate of dropouts from treatment as patients on long-term treatments would be better followed up. In the public system, this can be undertaken by the ASHA or ANM in the field, and can be monitored at the PHC by the medical officer.

Staff, too, need regular mentoring and nurturing. If public health facilities provide their staff opportunities to improve their knowledge and skills while at their place of posting, it may reduce staff absenteeism at the periphery. Satisfaction at work which is what most professionals desire, and the social capital generated, may offset the relatively low financial remunerations for a large section of doctors.

Medical colleges have a role beyond training undergraduate and postgraduate students and providing tertiary medical care. As illustrated by CMC, they can be a focus of continuing medical, nursing and paramedical training for the peripheral hospitals in the district, facilitate exchange programmes for peripheral doctors for short periods to an academic setting, and also provide specialist services to the periphery at regular intervals. The fact that in most states, the medical education and health services department function independent of each other is unfortunate.

Limited autonomy to government hospitals inhibits their creativity to respond to the need of the population. For example, strict governmental boundaries do not allow hospital staff to work in the periphery and for peripheral staff to work and learn in hospitals, both of which are critical to improving quality of health care. Providing greater autonomy to specific public sector hospitals would enable them to be more responsive to the needs of the people they serve.

The government's National Health Policy 2017[3] states as one of its objectives the progressive realization of universal health care. It aims to do this through providing free primary health-care services for all; providing secondary and tertiary care through a mix of provision through government facilities and purchasing some services in health-care deficit areas from private providers, preferably not-for-profit providers; and reducing catastrophic health expenditure. This will require adopting the policies of rationality and equity shown by the not-for-profit hospitals and regulating the insurance and the private health-care sector. The government may want to start by putting their own house in order by building transparency and accountability in its processes, reducing corruption and improving efficiency of services. Government hospitals should not set their criteria of quality by comparing themselves with the private sector or corporate hospitals, but should learn from the rights-based hospitals in the non-profit sector. It goes without saying that the public health system desperately needs the funding it has been deprived of for so long. The government can and should promote partnerships with private, not-for-profit hospitals, especially in rural areas, via funding and better relationship management—it should foster an attitude of trust and respect, rather than viewing these institutions with suspicion.

To sum up, secondary-level hospitals described here offer a model for providing responsive, low-cost and affordable care that is more urgently required in the public and private sector hospitals now than ever before. Significant increase in investment in public health facilities is urgent and long overdue. Relying on outsourcing secondary and tertiary health care through insurance schemes is insufficient and a waste of precious resources where the private and insurance sectors are so poorly regulated. A better health system is possible for all Indians with public health services, non-profits and the private sector working in tandem. What is required is the political will and the discipline to make it happen, and always by keeping the common citizen in mind.

Transforming Mental Health in India

Vikram Patel

Introduction

When people hear the words 'mental health', they instinctively think of mental illness. But mental health is much more than that; it is a valued personal asset. Indeed, mental health is defined by the World Health Organization as 'the capacity of thought, emotion and behaviour that enables every individual to realize their abilities in relation to their developmental stage, to cope with the stresses of life, to learn and work well and to make a contribution to their community'. The definition goes on to stress that 'mental health is an integral component of health and well-being and is more than the absence of mental disorder'. Mental health covers a range of human experiences, at the heart of which is the *trimurti* of thoughts, feelings and behaviours. Yet, we only become aware of our mental health when it is impaired.

Contrary to what biomedical systems have promoted, there is no clear dividing line between people with mental health problems (or 'disorders') and those without, because every aspect of human experience lies on a dimension, from positive at the one end to impaired at the other. Moreover, every 'symptom' of a mental health problem can also occur in perfectly reasonable and natural circumstances, such as feeling profound sadness at the loss of a loved one. In the absence of any biological marker of a mental health problem (the equivalent of a blood test for diabetes, for instance), we rely entirely on the person's subjective description of their mental health to arrive at a 'diagnosis' of whether they suffer from a mental health problem—by which we refer to a person who may benefit from clinical intervention like counselling or medication. In essence, virtually all mental health problems are manifestations of extremes of the *trimurti* of experiences in terms of their duration (usually at least continuously for two weeks), their pervasiveness (usually more than just one human experience) and their impact on daily life.

Based on clinical observations, biomedical science has identified a variety of mental health problems, which can afflict us at any point in our life course, although most begin before we reach our thirties. By far, the most common problems are those which affect our emotional states, such as depression and anxiety. It is the rarer ones, which affect our thoughts and behaviours, such as the psychoses, developmental disabilities and substance abuse, which are more devastating and associated with stigma and discrimination. This essay synthesizes what we know about mental health through this limited prism, the limitations of this approach, and how the pandemic presents a historic opportunity to transform our approach to mental health.

The Challenge

I write this essay as a sixth of the world's population battles a calamitous surge of the COVID-19 pandemic. Trauma swept across India in 2021 as millions of stories of suffering, despair and death twinned with profound helplessness, percolated into the consciousness of every person. The inevitable increase in experiences of anxiety, worry, hopelessness and anger were mostly rational responses of our minds to the extraordinary realities that we were facing. But it is inevitable that the increase in the prevalence of mental health distress across the population will fuel an increase in clinically significant mental disorders, adding to the large, unmet need for care that existed before the pandemic.

The government's National Mental Health Survey published in 2016 is the largest study of mental health undertaken in the country.[1] It reported that about one in ten adults was experiencing a clinically significant mental health problem (I suspect the prevalence would be similar in children), meaning that at least 100 million people in this country are affected at any point of time (and tens of millions more if one counts family members affected by mental health problems in a relative). Beyond these astonishing numbers, what was even more disturbing was that most of these persons, exceeding 90 per cent in the historically under-served rural and poorer communities of the country, had not received any treatment or care for their suffering.

The impact of this monumental unmet need for care, perhaps the largest across all health conditions, is profound and, for the most part, hidden from public view. In recent times, India has become the epicentre of global suicide mortality, accounting for about a quarter of all male and a third of all female suicide deaths. If suicide was an indicator of the loss of hope in one's future, then India is one of the most miserable countries in the world. It comes as no surprise, then, that India ranked near the bottom of the league of countries in the World Happiness Report 2020—alongside Afghanistan, South Sudan and Yemen. Pakistan, the neighbour we often look at with disdain, is seventy-eight ranks higher on the list; even Nepal, much poorer than us, is fifty ranks ahead. Indeed, we are the worst performer in the entire region. And what's more worrying is that our ranking on this index, built around a complex set of indicators including our economic strength, social support, levels of generosity and corruption, has been falling inexorably over the past five years, indicating grimmer times ahead. And this is before we even account for the pandemic.

A notable feature of the suicide mortality in India is that it is concentrated in young people; approximately two-thirds of all suicides occur in people under the age of thirty, and suicide is the leading cause of death in young Indians. To be sure, suicide is also a leading cause of death among young people in other countries. Youth is a vulnerable period for suicide globally because this is the phase of life characterized by unique neuro-developmental changes alongside dramatic transitions in one's self-image and aspirations, and this period is when some of the most important life decisions related to education and relationships are made. This is why suicide attempts by youth, unlike older adults, are often impulsive—triggered by acute disappointments such as a poor examination result or the loss of a romantic relationship. A curious observation is that the epicentres of suicide are in the more highly developed states of India, for example in the south of the country.[2] One may speculate that a key reason for this is the growing gap between the aspirations of educated youth, for example, to freely choose their life partner, and the reality of a harsh, inflexible and uncertain society in which they find themselves trying to find a footing.

Beyond suicide, the impact of mental health problems extends to reduced opportunities in education and employment, higher out-of-pocket expenditure on health care due to doctor-shopping for relief (including consulting other systems of medicine and religious providers), stress on caregivers and the pervasive effects of stigma. India also has to contend with the abuses of fundamental rights experienced by persons with severe and enduring mental health problems, in particular neuro-developmental disabilities and psychotic illness. The involuntary incarceration of persons with mental health problems in long-stay institutions, cut-off from their families and society, and often associated with profound indignities and violence, is a major source of the stigma attached to mental health problems and the consequent reluctance for people to seek help from mental health services.

The large unmet need for care for mental health problems can be attributed to both supply and demand side barriers. On the supply side, primary care physicians and other frontline providers have very little training or experience in mental health care. There are only about 10,000 specialist mental health professionals in the country, the vast majority of whom are concentrated in cities and big towns, and work in the private sector. Public expenditure on mental health is a miniscule 1 per cent of the overall health budget, which is itself one of the lowest in the world. Even this limited spending is entirely on hospital care and it is estimated that more than three-quarters of all inpatient beds for mental health care are situated in about forty large mental hospitals, most of which were built during the colonial era.

The District Mental Health Programme (DMHP) was initiated as one of the foundations of the National Mental Health Programme (NMHP) to provide mental health service at the community level by integrating mental health with the general health-care delivery system way back in 1982, making India one of the first low-income countries to adopt this goal. However, actual implementation of the programme was only initiated in four districts in 1996 and, on last count, this had been expanded to just 123 districts, a small fraction of the country.[3] Even in these few districts, the top-down, biomedical emphasis on psychiatry as the primary discipline of care has greatly limited impact, with most resources allocated to psychiatric outpatient clinics in the district hospital and occasional clinics in selected PHCs. The dominant interventions offered are medication, often in sub-optimal doses and durations. The lack of impact is vividly evidenced by the very low proportions of persons with mental health problems accessing care in the NMHS. Community-based mental health care, the most cost-effective and person-centred approach for mental health problems, is not available for any person in any part of the country. The supply-side barriers are even greater for specific groups in the population: especially children and adolescents (which is ironic as most mental health problems begin during this phase of life), for people with substance use problems and for older adults with dementia.

Demand-side barriers, apart from the obvious ones of cost, lack of access and poor quality of care, are related to the high levels of stigma associated with mental health problems and alienation from the narrow biomedical care model. This biomedical model is associated with the dominance of a care model which privileges the need for a diagnosis by a psychiatrist and the use of medication as the primary or only type of intervention. Unsurprisingly, these factors lead to large unmet needs for people with mental health problems which are 'hidden', such as mood and anxiety disorders, and childhood and adolescent mental health problems. Substance-use conditions, notably alcohol and opiate abuse, the latter presenting a major problem in some parts of the country, present a unique challenge: India is one of the handful of countries which continues to implement prohibition with stringent penalties, despite reams of evidence that this policy is ineffective, not only criminalizing a health problem but also fueling the criminal mafia which thrives on prohibition and deaths due to illegally brewed alcohols. The absence of alternative public health policies to address substance use instead of criminalizing the behaviour pushes the affected, in particular low-income individuals, to the margins of society.

The Opportunity

Several recent developments serve as foundations to reimagine and transform mental health care in India: the Mental Healthcare Act, community health worker delivered mental health care, and opportunities for prevention by acting on social determinants of mental health.

The Mental Health Care Act, 2016 radically transformed the legal basis of mental health care in India. There have been two previous mental health laws—the Indian Lunacy Act, 1912 and the Mental Health Act, 1987. The Indian Lunacy Act was primarily focused on protecting society from persons with mental illness, and its emphasis was on custodial care in institutions. The Lunacy Act presumed that persons with mental illness will spend the rest of their lives in such custodial institutions and the law focused on the rules for how people would be admitted to the hospital and the management of their property subsequent to their admission. The Mental Health Act, 1987 continued with certain regressive aspects of the Indian Lunacy Act, such as guardianship and the management of property of persons with mental illness, and was criticized for being largely concerned with regulation and administration of mental health care in institutional settings rather than addressing mental health problems of the community or protecting the rights of persons with mental illness.

At the heart of the new Mental Health Care Act are the twin rights of the person with mental illness to receive care and to live a life with dignity. The law recognizes the acute shortage and skewed distribution of mental health professionals and requires the government to put in place training programmes to achieve internationally accepted norms and, in the interim, to train all medical officers in public health facilities to provide basic and emergency mental health care. The law requires the government to provide a range of mental health services, including for those who have attempted suicide, from outpatient clinics to sheltered accommodation, through the public health sector in every district. The law aims for social inclusion of persons with mental illness by emphasizing that treatment and care is to be provided in a way that enables these persons to live with their families in their own community. The law introduces Advance Directives, which, like a living will, allows a person to state how they want to be treated if they are ever affected by a mental illness and not in a position to make decisions for themselves. The law requires parity of mental health services with physical health services, for example, in terms of provision of ambulance services, the quality of mental health facilities and the provision of medical insurance. Indeed, the new law is the first legislation in India enshrining the right to health care and the government's responsibility to fulfil this right, a goal which has remained elusive for the broader health aspirations of India's people.

The most innovative health-care delivery solution that has emerged from India is the reimagining of the human resource mix to address the enormous inequities in access to health care through 'task-sharing' with non-physician frontline providers. The deployment of over a million ASHA and other community health worker cadres in the past two decades, to deliver a range of health interventions, is one of the major contributors to the improvements in maternal and child health indicators in the country. Over the past decade, task-sharing has been adapted for the delivery of mental health interventions. Much of the science needed to design and evaluate this approach has been led by Sangath, a pioneering research organization headquartered in Goa, and working in several states of the country. A key element of Sangath's approach, in common with many other civil society organizations in the country (notable examples include the Banyan, the Mental Health Action Trust and the Indian Law Society's Centre for Mental Health Law and Policy) is the active engagement of community stakeholders to design, plan, deliver and hold mental health interventions accountable. One memorable example is that of the VISHRAM programme I led with Sangath in rural communities in Vidarbha, a region in the news because of farmer suicides, with the goal of addressing mental health problems, such as depression, which were strongly associated with suicide. A guiding principle of our effort was to work closely with grassroots organizations and community leaders to change the narrative on mental health and address the stigma associated with it. A key element of this revised narrative was to approach the subject of mental health problems through widely recognized social determinants, such as domestic violence and financial difficulties. VISHRAM led to a six-fold increase in demand for depression care, which included both community health worker-delivered psychosocial interventions and primary outpatient care, over a period of eighteen months.[4]

Sangath's research has demonstrated the effectiveness of community or lay health worker-delivered brief psychosocial interventions for the prevention and care of a range of mental health problems, from autism in childhood to emotional problems in adolescents to psychoses, depression and harmful drinking in adults. The global impact of Sangath's work is evidenced by the fact that one of its interventions, the Healthy Activity Program, a highly effective six-session psychological treatment for depression when delivered by lay counsellors,[5] has now been adapted for delivery in Canada and the USA—perhaps the only example of a mental health-care intervention developed in India being used in a wealthy country. Such innovations have redefined mental health care by affirming that the low-cost innovation of task-sharing mental health care is safe and effective. Thanks to this evidence, task-sharing is now recommended as the foundation of mental health care in national and global policy instruments, such as India's National Mental Health Policy and the WHO's Mental Health Action Plan.

A blind spot in mental health care has been the lack of attention to primary prevention despite compelling evidence of the role of social determinants in poor mental health. Many opportunities exist for prevention—targeting social determinants such as poverty, gender-based violence, quality education, community social capital and, most important of all, early life adversities such as child neglect and deprivation. We know what these strategies should be: promoting nurturing environments at home and schools, such as through parenting interventions and enhancing the school environment; cash transfers for low-income families; combating gender-based violence and other types of discrimination; and the building of life skills focused on social and emotional competencies in schools. Not only will these actions contribute to improving the population's mental health, they will help realize other major development priorities too.

While there has been a flourishing of initiatives to address this rising tide of mental health problems in response to the COVID-19 pandemic, most notably through telemedicine platforms, these suffer from the same barriers that have limited the equitable coverage of mental health care in the past: most rely on specialist providers, who are scarce in number. This is compounded by yet another barrier: digital literacy and adequate internet connectivity remain a distant goal for large swathes of our people, particularly amongst the poor and rural populations. Still, two aspects of telemedicine are particularly welcome. The first is the recognition of the opportunity for remote delivery, which can transform accessibility to specialist care in under-served regions as digital literacy and internet connectivity coverage increases. The second is the recognition of the value of psychological therapies, often ignored in mental health care and, at best, playing a poor cousin to medication options, as most mental health-care services on telemedicine platforms are provided by professionals who offer counselling interventions.

The Way Forward

Mental illnesses were already a leading cause of suffering and the most neglected health issue globally before the pandemic. The pandemic will, through worsening the social determinants of mental health, compound this crisis. Still, it also presents a unique and historic opportunity to reimagine mental health care, for its impact on mental health has been widely recognized and the inability of the existing mental health care system to respond to these needs fully exposed. This may well represent an opportune moment to mobilize the political will, resources, and community demand for scaling up the science which demonstrates the effectiveness of community and lay health worker-delivered psychosocial interventions for the prevention and care of mental health problems. Political will is needed not only to contribute materially, but also to support the engagement of a more diverse workforce to deliver mental health interventions and to empower persons with the lived experience to hold services accountable.

The 2018 Lancet Commission on Global Mental Health usefully laid down three key principles to reframe mental health.[6] These are all aligned with the guiding principles of India's Mental Health Care Act. First, we need to move beyond the narrow diagnosis-driven approach to classifying and labelling mental illness, an approach which may work well for infectious diseases but is ill-suited for mental health care, for reasons I have elaborated earlier, viz., that this approach is neither supported by decades of basic and epidemiological science, nor acceptable to communities globally. Offering mental health care must not be contingent on a 'diagnosis' and a diagnosis must not automatically mean the person needs to be 'treated' by a specialist mental health professional. Instead, the need of the hour is to build on the rich evidence on the effectiveness of frontline health worker-delivered low-cost psychosocial interventions to scale up the foundation of mental health care in the community.

That said, one size does not fit all for mental health care (as indeed, for any non-communicable health condition). There will always be persons who need more specialized care, including medications which can be transformative (think of antipsychotic drugs for schizophrenia or lithium for bipolar disorder) and brief hospital stays for acute crises. Even the much-maligned electroconvulsive therapy (ECT) has an important role when used judiciously for persons with severe and potentially life-threatening depression.[7] Thus, collaborative care, involving a close partnership between primary and community care providers, with mental health specialists working in tandem to help the person realize their desired outcomes (the hallmark of person-centred care), would comprise the best evidence-informed delivery model. This is, of course, the same delivery model for all chronic conditions, and offers an opportunity to integrate the care of physical and mental health concerns, bridging a chasm that has roots in the evolution of modern medicine. The integration of mental and physical health care is, arguably, a central vision of universal health coverage and the recent policy initiative to establish Health and Wellness Centres across the country is an ideal platform for such integrated, person-centred care.

Second, we need to reject once and for all the debate about whether mental health is determined by nurture or nature. A vast body of evidence clearly demonstrates that both play a role: a 'convergence' of genetic factors, early and contemporary life experiences, the social worlds which influence these experiences, and biological systems (ranging from neuro-developmental transitions to the gut microbiome) explains the mental health of each individual. Importantly, each of these domains includes both risk and protective factors and, given the enormous diversity in these domains, the sum of the permutations of factors across all domains is potentially infinite. This is yet another reason why the applications of categories of diagnoses are not acceptable as they fail to recognize the unique causal pathways for mental health problems that are deeply embedded in the personal life story of each individual. The final clinical picture captured in a diagnosis tells us nothing about this personal story.

A convergent approach emphasizes the role of social determinants, in particular in the first two decades of life when the brain is most responsive to environmental influences, and recognizes the importance of nurturing environments at home, in schools, in neighbourhoods, in society and, increasingly, in the digital space in promoting mental health and preventing mental illness. Much of the effort to address prevention will lie outside the health sector, for instance, with the ministries concerned with Women & Child Development or Education, indicating the importance of inter-sectoral partnerships for mental health.

Third, we need to reframe mental health through the lens of human rights. Three specific kinds of rights are particularly relevant. The first is the right to be protected from known harms which adversely affect mental health, in particular adversities in childhood, violence through the life course, any form of discrimination, and the damaging effects on mental health of living in conditions of poverty. Second is the right to receive care, on par with any other health condition and regardless of the ability to pay for treatment of a mental health condition. Third, and most important of all, is the right to the freedom to choose what type of care, if any, a person wishes to receive, without any coercion or fear. This right is aligned with the UN Convention for the Rights of Persons with Disability's vision of equality for persons with psychosocial disability on all matters, including the right to refuse treatment for a health condition. The Mental Health Care Act requires the regulatory provision of District Boards, consisting of a district judge, psychiatrist and users and caregivers, to ensure that the rights of persons with mental health problems are respected when they receive care. This is one major step towards realizing the goal of supported decision-making, a strategy to enable a person with a mental health problem make a decision about treatment which is in their own interest. This would replace the existing approach of decision-making being substituted through a legal process, for example to the judgement of a psychiatrist or magistrate.

There are a number of examples of how these three principles have been operationalized in India, but most are primarily research or demonstration projects (Box 1); a key task now is to scale up the science and opportunities by building a diverse coalition of actors across sectors who are united in the goal of realizing the vision of the Mental Health Care Act. These actions will need to unleash the power of communities, through building a community-based workforce for delivering mental health interventions, mobilizing political will and resources for scaling up, enabling access to specialized mental health services for those who need such care, and holding mental health services accountable. This effort should especially focus on the empowerment of persons with the lived experience of mental health problems, who must not face exclusion or discrimination in any sector of society, notably education, employment and civil rights. Their engagement is also critical for addressing the stigma and discrimination associated with mental illness, for social contact with persons with lived experience is the most effective strategy to address the barriers to inclusion and parity. The recognition of the inseparable association of mental health with social determinants demands actions at the structural level, for example cash transfers to alleviate acute indebtedness and supporting low-income families to offer nurturing environments to young children. Opportunities to integrate mental health with other health and social programmes, such as for non-communicable diseases and adolescent health, should be encouraged. Initiatives which encourage people to disclose their mental health problems, for example the www.itsoktotalk.in which targets young people, could help reduce the stigma associated with seeking care. And we must never lose sight on ensuring equitable coverage of care for persons who are more vulnerable to suffer mental health problems, such as those who live in conditions of extreme deprivation or who face social exclusion and violence.

Case Studies of Initiatives to Transform Mental Health Care in India

Empowering community-based frontline providers to deliver evidence-based mental health care: EMPOWER (www.empower.care) is an innovative programme which seeks to build the mental health workforce through using a suite of connected technologies to enable frontline providers (for example community health workers) to learn, deliver and master evidence-based, brief psychosocial interventions. Foundational work has been conducted by Sangath in Madhya Pradesh, where training to deliver the Healthy Activity Programme (a brief psychological treatment for depression) has been digitized (in Hindi) and tested with ASHAs. Scaling up of this intervention has now begun in three districts and adaptations for other states (e.g., Gujarat) and the development of digital tools for peer supervision and quality assurance is in progress.

Fostering nurturing environments for children and adolescents: The SEHER intervention was designed by Sangath to promote school 'climate', targeting the social environment in schools, including elements such as social, emotional and physical safety, through the active engagement of students. The multi-component intervention was designed through a participatory process and then evaluated in a cluster randomized controlled trial in seventy-four schools in Bihar. The intervention showed large benefits, when coordinated by a lay counsellor, on school climate, mental health and violence outcomes. SEHER is now being adapted and implemented in three diverse contexts: in schools in the city of Pimpri-Chinchwad (Maharashtra); urban and rural schools in Karnataka; and Ashramshalas, a residential school setting for underprivileged children, in Gadchiroli district (Maharashtra).

A rights-based approach for vulnerable persons with serious mental illness: The Banyan works with vulnerable populations with the experience of homelessness, social disadvantage and mental health challenges and has serviced a million low-income households since its inception in 1993 in Tamil Nadu. The Banyan has expanded its reach to wider sections of disadvantaged communities, providing comprehensive, culturally sensitive and person-centred mental health and social care services through its flagship programmes—

the Emergency Care and Recovery Centre (ECRC) that offers crisis support and 'Home Again' that offers long-term inclusive living options. Additionally, the Centre for Social Needs and Livelihoods facilitates social entitlements, livelihoods and continued mental health-care access, inspiring social mixing and focus on participation. The Banyan has scaled its ECRC Model across ten districts in Tamil Nadu and is in the process of further scaling up to all thirty-seven districts, while also scaling up 'Home Again' in districts in ten states in India and Sri Lanka.

In the spirit of the Sustainable Development Goals, the moral imperative for mental health care is to leave no one behind by implementing evidence-informed community delivered programmes for the care and prevention of mental health problems, embedded in a universal health coverage and empowerment framework. Investing in such a reformed mental health system can enable individuals to regain hope for the future and the necessary cognitive and emotional capabilities to be effective in their work and personal lives and to participate meaningfully in their social world. Collectively, it can help build stronger, more cohesive communities, improving their capacities to confront not only pandemics but also the economic and ecological crises that loom in our post-pandemic future. Ultimately, we need to recognize and celebrate mental health as a fundamental, universal human quality, an indivisible part of health important to all people in all communities, and care for which should be regarded as a national public good.

People over Profits: Reshaping India's Private Health Care

Abhay Shukla, Shweta Marathe and Kanchan Pawar

'We thus find ourselves at a crossroads: health care can be considered a commodity to be sold, or it can be considered a basic social right. It cannot comfortably be considered both of these at the same time. This, I believe, is the great drama of medicine at the start of this century. And this is the choice before all people of faith and good will in these dangerous times.'

—Paul Farmer[1]

Introduction: Reality of the Private Health-Care Sector in India

One chronic illness or unexpected health emergency is enough to wipe out all the savings of a family and incur a lifetime of debt and poverty. Unfettered by regulations on price or quality of services, the dizzying growth of the for-profit private health-care sector in the past three decades in India has resulted in the formation of a powerful medical industrial complex comprising of corporate, multi-specialty private hospitals, private medical colleges, pharmaceutical and medical devices industry, and diagnostic chains, which stonewall most attempts for regulation by the state that are perceived to threaten their profit margins.

The health-care system in India is indeed a study in contradictions. We rank fifth on the Global Medical Tourism Index due to our pool of highly experienced and skilled doctors working in state-of-the-art private hospitals, but rank 145th among 195 countries on the Global Healthcare Quality and Access Index.[2, 3] India is a global leader in the manufacture of low-cost generic drugs, but a majority of our citizens cannot afford life-saving medicines.

The story of how India's private health-care sector has flourished is a direct corollary of decades of neglect and underinvestment in India's public health system, along with active encouragement of privatization and fervent espousal of neoliberal reforms since the 1990s, which increasingly promoted commercialization of health care. Though health has been acknowledged as being fundamental to national progress, public spending on health in India has never reflected this priority, with successive governments investing less than 1 per cent of the country's gross domestic product (GDP) over most of the past seven decades. At the national level, governments are presently investing barely 1.2 per cent of GDP on public health, which is far below the average for lower-middle income countries (2.4 per cent) and upper-middle-income countries (3.8 per cent).[4]

According to business reports, the health-care sector in India has become an attractive site for private capital investment by global investment firms, private equity funds, high-net-worth-individuals, and also by global financial institutions such as the International Finance Corporation (IFC). Foreign investment in the hospital sector in India increased from merely Rs 31 crore in 2001–02, to Rs 3995 crore in 2013–14,[5] an over hundred-fold increase in little more than a decade. Several Indian multinational health-care companies have a growing presence in neighbouring South Asian countries, as well as in the Gulf and in some African countries, and have been listed on stock exchanges to access additional capital to finance their expansion.[6] This influx of capital has resulted in a burgeoning corporate health-care sector, fuelling the corporatization of health care in India.

In most states, the overstretched public health sector leaves people with no option but to seek health care from the private sector. Data from the National Sample Survey Office 75th round conducted in 2017–18 shows that 70 per cent of all patients are treated in the private health-care sector, while 58 per cent of all inpatients are hospitalized in private hospitals. The private sector engages 90 per cent of all allopathic doctors.[7] In a country where just 15 per cent of the population is covered by insurance, 68 per cent of total expenditure on health care is paid out of pocket, as compared to a world average of 18.2,[8] with 43 per cent of this out-of-pocket expenditure being on medicines alone.[9] Hence, it is hardly surprising to know that an estimated 55 million Indians are pushed below the poverty line every year due to catastrophic health-care expenses. With private hospitals keen to maximize profits at any costs, vulnerable people seeking health care are prescribed unwarranted treatment and presented with unduly high health-care bills.[10] Women have been disproportionately affected by profiteering: subjected to unnecessary hysterectomies[11] and caesarean sections[12] in private hospitals, which often spill over into publicly funded insurance schemes involving private providers.

While the corporate captains of commercialization remain out of reach of popular accountability, unfortunate incidents of verbal and physical violence against health-care professionals are on the rise across India, as people round on hapless frontline service providers. People have now begun to express their inchoate sense of anger and frustration with a private health-care sector that often exploits them financially when they are most vulnerable, largely denies them redressal in the case of medical negligence and malpractice, and tends to one-sidedly protect hospitals and doctors from the consequences of their actions. A profession once revered is now increasingly reviled, as an increasingly vocal population airs its grievances on social media and shares proof of exorbitant bills and medical malpractice.

Need for Regulation and Socialization

The Clinical Establishment Act (CEA) was passed in 2010 by the Union government, to introduce standards of quality, and to regulate the cost of health care in private health-care facilities across India. Even though the Act has been adopted by eleven states and six union territories, its effective implementation based on permanent registration of establishments is still pending ten years later, due to stiff resistance from the private medical lobby. Health services being a state subject, implementation of a uniform regulatory framework ensuring price control and standardized protocols in health care is a challenge no government has yet fully succeeded in tackling, primarily due to the vested interests and political influence of the medical industrial complex. Repeatedly hit by claims of corruption, the now defunct Medical Council of India failed in its function of self-regulation by the medical profession, and ended as an example of regulatory capture, controlled by sections of the very profession it was supposed to regulate, with state medical councils faring no better.[13]

In this essay, we begin with a description of the differentiated nature of the private sector in India. We briefly outline the evolution of the private sector since 1950 and point to the internal contradictions of private health-care sector linked with corporatization of health care. We then analyse how the private sector lacks effective regulation and its consequences for society, which have been strikingly exposed during the COVID-19 pandemic. We also examine lessons from the COVID-19 epidemic regarding regulation of private health care, suggesting the need for re-imagining public engagement of private health care. Finally, we deliberate on institutionalized mechanisms for regulation and socialization of private health care towards attaining UHC while providing reference to illustrative examples from a couple of countries.

Differentiated Nature and Internal Contradictions of Private Health-Care Sector

While we analyze the current role of the private health-care sector, it is pertinent to recognize its extremely heterogeneous nature. The private health-care sector in India is comprised of a vast range of providers such as formal and informal, for-profit and not-for-profit, family investment-based and for-profit corporation, small, medium and large entities. These services are further classified, viz., hospitals, medical and nursing homes, dental care practices, physiotherapists, diagnostic and pathological laboratories, blood banks and others, which include independent ambulatory care, Ayurveda, Unani and homoeopathy practitioners. While medical pluralism with respect to medical systems exists, according to data on the composition of doctors[14] in India, the private health-care sector is highly dominated by allopathic doctors with a share of 77.2 per cent, whereas the shares of homoeopathy and Ayurveda doctors is noted to be around 8.1 per cent, and 13.5 per cent respectively.

The evolution of the private health-care sector in India can be broadly outlined in three phases. In its first phase (1950s–70s), the health-care sector was mostly comprised of socially embedded institutions—public or charitable hospitals, along with individual private practitioners often working as family doctors—whose primary logic consisted of responding to health-care needs of the people they served. The second phase (1980s–2000s) witnessed the first wave of commercialization penetrating all spheres of society, coupled with the neoliberal policy framework giving a boost to commercialization of health care. There was a rise of private nursing homes and smaller private hospitals; health care was being converted into a market-based commodity, and profit-making emerged as an important dynamic. This created the ground for the post-millennium third phase (2000s onwards) with growing corporatization, wherein large private and corporate hospitals have emerged as significant players, whose overwhelming driving logic is the maximization of profits. This transition is evident from NSSO data as well, which shows a declining trend in individual-run enterprises in the private health sector between 2001–02 and 2010–11, and an increasing trend towards small-, medium- and large-sized enterprises. Further, this data also shows the steep growth in number of for-profit entities. At the time of Independence, around 21.4 per cent of private health enterprises registered themselves as not-for-profit entities (NPE). By 2010-11, the NPE share had fallen to around 1.6 per cent. Today, most enterprises (about 98.4 per cent) are for-profit (FPE) in nature.[15] In the latest phase of commercialization of health care, the process of the corporatization of health care is related to but not limited to corporate hospitals. It is also strongly influencing and reshaping other players in the sector in various ways—including individual practitioners, charitable private hospitals, diagnostic centres and even pharmacies.

With such developments, internal contradictions within the private health-care sector are apparent. Overall, corporatized health care has converted the health sector in India from its earlier mould of socially embedded institutions, to becoming an arena for aggressive maximization of profits. Polarization seems to be underway in the private health-care sector, with individual doctor-run smaller hospitals and nursing homes facing the heat of competition by well-funded and equipped, profit-centred corporate and large private hospitals. Many nursing homes, small hospitals and hitherto not-for-profit hospitals have closed down across the country. The remaining are faced with the threat of extinction, and to escape this fate, they are emulating corporate hospital management styles. This includes adopting their marketing practices and incentivizing doctor's performances in terms of referrals, billable procedures and tests, with a focus on maximizing profits. Indian and multinational health-care funds are taking over and merging hospitals in cities. Several companies have tied up with for-profit hospitals and trust hospitals for the management of their hospital services.

A recent case study from Maharashtra on corporatization and its impacts,[16] has reported on the implications of corporatization of private health care for other types of clinical establishments. The study mentions how low- and medium-budget private nursing homes are a 'dying phenomenon' in cities and towns. The same study also highlights the tensions felt by medical professionals about opportunities and challenges in the contemporary health-care system. The emergence of corporate management in hospitals has changed the doctor–hospital relationship, since their employment as consultants is often conditional on fulfilment of performance targets. The pressure to make profits for the hospital puts constraints on the professional autonomy of doctors and contributes to cost inflation while promoting medical malpractice and loss of trust in doctor–patient relationships. Nurses and other health-care staff in private hospitals also often face the brunt of low wages, hire-and-fire policies and onerous working conditions. These internal tensions within the private health-care sector need to be recognized while conceptualizing directions for change.

Lack of Effective Regulation Leading to Market Failure

Given that India is currently quite dependent on the private health-care sector, the lack of effective regulation and standardization has widespread consequences which affect every segment of society. The Government of India has been receiving many complaints[17] regarding malpractices in private clinical establishments, particularly large multi-specialty hospitals and corporate establishments. Patients admitted in hospitals are often forced to avail of in-house diagnostics services and to purchase medicines, consumables and implants from select vendors. These are sold with hefty profit margins ranging from 100 per cent to 1737 per cent according to a study by the National Pharmaceutical Pricing Authority (NPPA), Government of India.[18] Lack of Standard Treatment Protocols leads to widespread irrational and unnecessary treatments, tests and procedures. Vulnerable patients and their families complain about lack of transparency in treatment, of medical negligence, violation of the patients' rights and the frustration of facing an opaque and biased system of redressal, which often does not give them justice.

The health-care sector is disproportionately prone to market failure, which can only be curbed by effective and comprehensive regulation in public interest. It has long been recognized across the world that the delivery of health care should not be organized as a purely commercial activity, dictated by the market. The Nobel Prize-winning economist Kenneth Arrow[19] had warned over half a century ago that in the realm of health care, competitive markets generate inefficient allocation of resources, leading to market failures; non-market institutions are necessary to compensate for these. Policymakers in India have nevertheless conveniently turned a blind eye to this lesson over the last several decades. Here it is relevant to note that without ensuring mechanisms for effective regulation of private health care, the Union government launched the Ayushman Bharat-Pradhan Mantri Jan Arogya Yojana (AB-PMJAY) in 2018, an insurance scheme covering costs of secondary and tertiary care up to Rs 5 lakh for 10.74 crore of India's poorest families, based on the public-private partnership (PPP) model for provision of health care.

Now more than ever, regulation of health care cannot be just left to groups of private medical professionals who dominate medical councils. The reasons for their inability to self-regulate is evident.[20] Strong stewardship by state institutions, combined with effective frameworks for social accountability are necessary to reinstate the 'social' logic, which must prevail over the dominant 'profit' logic in the contemporary health system. Effective regulation, social accountability, and transparent governance regarding private health-care providers are key steps to ensure that health care moves in the direction of becoming a public good, free from the dictates of commercialization.

Lessons from the COVID-19 Epidemic Regarding Regulation of the Private Health-Care Sector

The COVID-19 epidemic has underscored some of the major problems related to the private health-care sector in India, but has also offered reason for modest hopes regarding possibilities of regulation of the private health-care sector. The limited capacities of the public health system prompted several Indian states to take unconventional and unprecedented steps for mandatory engagement of the private health-care sector to meet the public health emergency. In response to reports of certain private hospitals evicting[21] patients with COVID-19 symptoms, as well as reducing or shutting down their outpatient and inpatient services, some states responded by rapidly issuing orders for requisitioning private health-care providers.

Several complaints were reported of hospitals overcharging for COVID-19 tests and treatment in different parts of the country, with some corporate hospitals and diagnostic chains capitalizing on the opportunity to charge patients exorbitant COVID-care packages. In response to a large number of grievances of overcharging during the pandemic, it is quite notable that around fifteen Indian states directed private hospitals to regulate rates. Further, various states either converted private hospitals into designated COVID-19 care centres or took over the private hospitals for COVID-19 care. Maharashtra also declared that coverage of the Mahatma Phule Jeevandayi Arogya Yojana (MPJAY), the state health insurance scheme for secondary and tertiary health care for lower-income groups, would be extended to all its residents.

According to a 2021 decision by the Union Health Ministry, existing packages in PM-JAY for pneumonia, respiratory failure and other conditions could be used for COVID-19 patients. However, there was considerable evidence that many PMJAY-enrolled private hospitals were not fulfilling the expectation of providing free care to COVID patients.[22]

Despite state measures, many private hospitals indulged in exploitative and unethical practices—such as exorbitant charges, non-transparency in treatment and billing, not informing patients about rate regulation and public schemes, forcing patients to pay hefty advances and denying admission without advance payment—at the cost of affordability, rational care and access to care for large sections of the population. In Pune alone, 1387 complaints of overcharging were received from August 2020 to July 2020.[23] In light of this, in many cities, state governments promptly issued a show-cause notice to private hospitals for flouting the state orders and alleged refusal of beds for patients. The municipal corporations of Mumbai and Pune conducted audits to detect inflated bills and prevent overcharging by private hospitals. During the second wave of the pandemic, around seventy auditors were put on the job in Mumbai. A suo motu audit of around 11,000 bills generated during December 2020 to April 2021 was done and a total of Rs 157.5 million was reduced or refunded by hospitals.[24] In Pune too, two teams of auditors were deployed and refunded Rs 64.4 million to patients.[25]

These examples demonstrate how certain governments took exceptional measures to implement mandatory engagement of the private sector for COVID-19 related care and adopt new forms of engagement; these, for a change, were much more on the terms set by the public system than the private sector. An issue as contentious and disputed as rate regulation became feasible, albeit to a limited extent, during this unprecedented public health emergency because public interest and social obligation for the provision of health care became paramount. The political will of governments for regulated engagement of private providers seems to have surfaced as a response to people's demand for affordable health care in a public health crisis, overcoming long-standing resistance of the private health-care lobby.

These exceptional measures can be viewed as a potential precedent for the state to reclaim its shrinking role in health sector governance while effectively regulating the private health-care sector. Notwithstanding its widespread negative impacts, the COVID-19 epidemic has shown a silver lining in terms of opening the way for re-imagining public engagement of private health care and building a wider framework of public obligation and social accountability of the private sector, driven by the public health system.

Civic Action for Social Accountability of Private Health Care

The past decade has witnessed growing support and activism among civil society organizations and ordinary citizens in India for building accountability of the private health-care sector and protection of Patient's Rights. Networks like Jan Swasthya Abhiyan (People's Health Movement–India) seek to mainstream the discourse on social accountability of the private health-care sector. Books such as *Dissenting Diagnosis* (Gadre and Shukla, 2016) and *Healers & Predators—Healthcare Corruption in India* (Nundy, Desiraju and Nagral, 2018), authored by senior health-care professionals disturbed by the increasing commercialization of medicine in India, are powerful 'insider' accounts of prevailing corruption, malpractices and profiteering in the private health sector in India. These books have initiated a debate on the reality of commercialized medical practice and have motivated sections of ethical doctors to come together to advocate for accountability in the private health-care sector through various platforms.[26]

Civil society networks have supported citizen activists like lawyer Birender Sangwan, who filed a PIL in the Supreme Court to regulate the price of exorbitantly expensive cardiac stents in

2014, leading the National Pharmaceutical Pricing Authority to bring down stent prices by over 70 per cent in 2017.[27] The family of patient-victim Adya Singh, who tragically lost her life after treatment in a large corporate hospital accompanied by grossly inflated bills, has started an organization called All India Patients' Rights Group. Such voices are strengthening the impetus for regulation of the private health-care sector in India.

Examples of Socially Regulated Health-Care Systems from Other Countries

Keeping this socio-political background in view and the heightened interest in the functioning of health systems in the wake of the COVID-19 epidemic, Central and state governments should build on this momentum to introduce regulatory measures in the private health sector as they move towards progressive realization of the Right to Healthcare.

Efforts to regulate the private health sector so far, which primarily use a formalistic 'enforcement' approach, have been consistently stymied by the medical lobby, thus proving that while such an approach may work to regulate other economic sectors, it does not work well for health care, due to factors such as the inherent information and power asymmetry between patient and provider. In fact, health care should not be treated as a market commodity, and instead must be increasingly regarded as a public good which would be available to all, free of cost at point of service.

There are precedents for this, as socially regulated health-care systems providing universal access to health care are a norm in some rich and developed nations such as Austria, Norway, Japan and Austria. In Japan, the estimated total health expenditure amounts to approximately 11 per cent of GDP, of which 84 per cent is publicly financed, mainly through its Statutory Health Insurance System (SHIS), funded by taxes and individual contributions through employment-based or residence-based health insurance plans. The national government regulates nearly all aspects of the SHIS; it sets the SHIS fee schedule for all primary and specialist services and gives subsidies to local governments, insurers and providers. It also establishes and enforces detailed regulations for insurers and health providers. It is notable that only non-profit entities are allowed to run hospitals in Japan, in effect shielding health care from profit-making business practices, despite Japan being a hardcore capitalist country. Though most care is provided by private-owned clinics and hospitals, providers are prohibited from balance billing.[28]

Though the costs of a universal health-care system pose a challenge to developing countries, which have large populations of non-tax paying citizens, in recent years, Thailand has been hailed as an example of how collective commitment to universal health care in lower-middle income countries can result in successful implementation of reforms towards that end. Starting in 2001, Thailand implemented a universal coverage scheme (UCS) funded through general taxation to provide health care to an estimated 75 per cent of its population (47 million people) who are not covered by its Social Security Scheme (SSS) for private sector employees (16 per cent) and Civil Servant Medical Benefit Scheme (CSMBS) for government employees (9 per cent). The scheme has enabled provision of a comprehensive health package of essential health services that is free at point of service to all Thai citizens, resulting in a significant drop in catastrophic health expenditure and out-of-pocket payment over the past decade, increased access to health care services and improved health parameters.[29]

The UCS scheme succeeded due to Thailand's long-term investment in public health infrastructure and health workforce, particularly in rural areas over five decades. The country's current health expenditure is 3.8 per cent of its GDP. All public health facilities are a part of UCS, while private health sector involvement is still limited, with private hospitals catering to a mere estimated 6 per cent of all beneficiaries.[30] The government has leveraged the large scale of UCS to procure generic drugs and health services at lower costs.

Directions for Change: Steps for Regulation and Socialization of Private Health Care

If private resources are to be harnessed for public good, then the state may have to consider moving beyond formalistic 'enforcement' and instead using an 'interventionist' approach towards regulation. This would restructure the market to align with national health goals and priorities, while ensuring accountability of the private health sector with a mix of legal, financial and social regulatory tools. Regulation of the private health-care sector should include the following measures in the near future:

1. Effective implementation of the Clinical Establishment Act, 2010, and similar state-specific legislations after notifying Minimum Standards. This should include regulation of rates, transparency in pricing and compliance with Standard Treatment Protocols applicable to all health-care institutions.
2. Mechanisms to enable health-care professionals and facilities to comply with regulations, through:
    *   adopting a differential approach and providing additional support to smaller, rural and genuinely not-for-profit health-care establishments;
    *   awareness and capacity building of providers, especially in the initial stages, to overcome their distrust and biases in public regulation;
    *   providing some transition time to meet infrastructure and human resource standards, depending on their category and ability to meet costs of regulatory compliance.
3. Implementation of the Patient Rights Charter in all public and private hospitals, along with establishing patient-friendly grievance redressal mechanisms at hospital, state and national

levels for victims of medical negligence and malpractice, which are committed to timely and fair resolution of disputes.

4. Staffing regulatory agencies with adequate human power and resources, building their institutional capacity to implement and monitor regulations.

5. Ensuring that the regulatory agency responsible for developing health care prices in the private sector will adjust them for fairness (keeping in view geographical cost adjustments, need to ensure health care access to under-served populations etc.)[31] and revise them periodically. The government should also ensure that stakeholders like medical associations can provide feedback and give inputs in the price setting process, to avoid potential stalemate situations.

6. Promoting social accountability through creation of multi-stakeholder governance platforms at all levels of governance including district, state and national levels. These would be representative of key stakeholders and should include patient groups, civil society organizations working on health rights, health workers' associations, women's organizations, as well as associations of medical professionals. Such participatory governance of health systems will ensure equitable access to health-care services, minimize malpractice due to monitoring of performance and ensure that all stakeholders have a voice at the table.

Such an approach of 'social regulation' would have three interrelated components: *State regulation*, based on law and authorities; *multi-stakeholder accountability and oversight bodies*, including civil society, patients' groups and medical professionals to monitor regulatory and grievance redressal processes; and *technical elements of self-regulation*, such as standard treatment protocols to be developed by bodies of diverse health-care professionals, including public and not-for-profit health experts. This kind of regulatory design should be evolved through participatory processes and consultations, rather than purely administrative diktat or 'captured' regulatory design dominated by the private sector lobby.

Further, the regulatory framework involving private health-care providers should extend beyond merely streamlining the market (limited to current 'enforcement' type regulation, mostly focused on physical standards). Instead, the process of regulation needs to be combined with a powerful movement to bring large sections of the private health-care sector under public stewardship and social control, while using public funding as an influential lever. It would also be insufficient to rely on optional, contractual obligations of private providers with current publicly funded health insurance schemes, since these depend purely on the wish of the providers, who have the freedom to opt out of such schemes if terms and conditions are perceived as being unfavourable. Examples of denial of care in private hospitals to insured people during the COVID-19 epidemic has illustrated the limited efficacy of the current commercial insurance-based model.

Today, corporatized health care is straining for further markets, seeking to fill unoccupied beds in hospitals, but is constrained by the limited purchasing capacity of the majority of population. In this scenario, two possibilities are emerging. The first scenario, which is currently unfolding, is of corporate and large private health-care providers turning to the state to fuel their next phase of expansion—based on large-scale state subsidization through health insurance schemes. Further growth of PM-JAY and state-specific health insurance schemes, handing over not only secondary and tertiary but also possibly primary health-care provisioning to corporate chains would characterize this trajectory.

However, the State can intervene quite differently for an alternative scenario—with the development of a public-centred Universal Health Care system. This would reverse the trend of corporatization by strengthening public health provisioning, partly socializing large numbers of individual and smaller providers, and confining corporate providers to narrow elite market segments, thus moving towards an overall de-commodified health-care system.

In contrast to the current health insurance scheme-based approaches, the approach to engagement of private health sector should be through regulated involvement of majority of private providers in a publicly managed and funded Universal Health Care system. Here engagement of private providers would be organized in a manner that would complement and strengthen public health services. This could be done by contracting entire private hospitals wherever possible, or a majority of beds in private hospitals above a specified minimum size, for supporting the publicly organized health-care system. Individual private physicians could also be insourced to provide outpatient health services in underserved remote and rural areas, thus improving access to care. Such arrangements would add to the capacity of the public health system and would fill the gaps in public health provisioning, while providing tax-funded free and quality health care to all. Over time, private providers would be increasingly 'socialized' and made to function as an extension of the public system. Such providers would be held socially accountable just like public health services, with Right to Information, community-based monitoring and grievance redressal being applicable to all providers, and enforced through participatory mechanisms.

Governments should use pricing and payment systems that ensure fair and timely reimbursement for services provided by private sector health-care providers as powerful incentives to deliver quality care and to improve efficiency. When the state becomes by far the biggest purchaser of health-care services, not only can it dictate terms but also overcome entrenched resistance to regulation, by requiring compliance with standards and rationality of care as a precondition for purchase of services.

Further, given the considerable popularity and usage of AYUSH (Ayurveda, Yoga and Naturopathy, Unani, Siddha and Homoeopathy) systems of healing, it is important that any proposed

UHC system include plans to integrate and promote these systems. Historically, AYUSH systems of medicine, including traditional healers, have been on the whole more socially embedded than biomedicine, and have also been less affected by corporatization. However, now commercialization and associated malpractices are affecting some practitioners of these systems too. This needs to be checked by providing AYUSH systems greater public funding and support, combined with appropriate forms of regulation. While including AYUSH systems in the UHC system, we can start with an approach of health-care pluralism, where AYUSH systems could be made available to people as a choice at various levels, and practitioners will be enabled to practise their system along with its theoretical framework, clinical diagnosis, and validation methods. This should progressively move towards 'integrated health care', whereby these forms of healing are integrated into UHC systems, while using evidence-based protocols. These would make available biomedical treatment as well as specific AYUSH measures in synergistic manner, in ways which could provide the maximum benefit to the patient, including possible integrated care regimens.

Such integrated efforts to expand and strengthen public provisioning, along with regulated involvement of a reformed private health-care sector, can create much-needed momentum towards ensuring Universal Health Care, which will help us to realize the India of our dreams.

Redesigning and Revitalizing India's Public Health Governance: Addressing Abiding Antagonisms

T. Sundararaman and Mekhala Krishnamurthy

Introduction

India, with its particular history of chronic underinvestment in public health, has experienced a long process of passive privatization which has produced a system characterized by incredibly high levels of out-of-pocket expenditure and persistently poor health outcomes. That this has taken place in spite of a seemingly dense institutional landscape with a wide range of public health institutions has only intensified the lack of confidence in the state and its capacity to deliver at all levels.

From Abiding Antagonism to Shared Ownership and Accountability

Yet, state capacity is not a one-time endowment but a continuous process of institutional evolution. Moreover, strong public institutions are not alternatives but prerequisites for shaping and sustaining comprehensive and equitable health systems. This will not be achieved by simply defending the state and public system, as it currently exists. It requires us to identify and understand the old and emerging fault lines upon which institutions are erected, become entrenched and are undermined over time. This essay identifies two of the most critical, enduring and unresolved sources of institutional tension and antagonism in the field of health in India: the dynamic between the Centre and the states and the relationship between the 'technical' and the 'administrative'. The first is—literally and figuratively—a *constitutional* question at the heart of Indian federalism. The second, the tension between the technical and the administrative, constitutes the very field of public health itself, whether in India or anywhere else.

These foundational antagonisms have made it difficult to fix accountability and have enabled a constant passing of the proverbial buck between different levels and 'wings' of the system. Engaging deeply with the existing realities of the present system, its deep infirmities and varied endowments, they must be addressed in a way that is both grounded and imaginative if we are to begin to redesign and revitalize the ecosystem of public health institutions in India. This essay is a modest effort towards such engagement.

It begins by briefly laying out the institutional landscape governing health, before considering various aspects of the Centre–state balance and the complex and contested relationship between technical experts and generalist administrators in shaping institutional capacity for public health and health systems in India. The essay then briefly examines the design and contribution of knowledge management institutions. Each section suggests ways in which the challenges might be reframed and addressed.

The Current Structure of Governance

Currently, at the Centre, all aspects of health are largely under the Ministry of Health and Family Welfare. AYUSH services, pharmaceuticals and certain aspects of financing of private-sector services like health insurance and foreign direct investment are the exceptions. One new administrative structure that was established in January 2019 and is outside the health ministry is the National Health Authority, the implications of which we will discuss in a later section.

The Ministry of Health and Family Welfare is accountable to Parliament, which sanctions its budget and to which the ministry reports annually. The minister appointed by the elected government is the chief executive. The Parliament legislates and also exercises oversight over the functioning of the ministry. Detailed discussions take place through its Standing Parliamentary Committee on Health. To help this committee in its assessment, the Office of Comptroller General of Accounts submits its reports, as do other review bodies and commissions.

The Union ministry is made up of two departments with separate secretaries—one for health research and the other for all other aspects. The Office of the Directorate General of Health Services (DGHS) is the main technical adviser in the Department of Health and Family Welfare. More than fifteen apex public health institutions provide support, some of which report directly to the Secretary and some through the DGHS.

In terms of coordination with states, there are many programme-specific mechanisms, but the Council of Health and Family Welfare (CHFW) is the formal institution created to fulfil the mandate under Article 263 (on inter-state coordination) of the Constitution. The Union Minister for Health and Family Welfare is chairperson, while the Minister of State for Health & Family Welfare is the vice-chairperson. Member, NITI Aayog and Ministers for Health & Family Welfare, Medical Education and Public Health in the States/Union Territories, representatives of Union Territories, four Members of Parliament, six non-officials and eleven eminent individuals are members.

Health Care and the Centre–State Balance

The Constitutional Mandate

Under the Constitution, much of health care—preventive, promotive and curative—belongs to the state list, that is, only states have jurisdiction over the subject. This is articulated as 'public health and sanitation, hospitals and dispensaries'. However, population control and family planning, the spread of communicable disease, drugs, medical education, universities and professional bodies, vital statistics, including the registration of births and deaths, food adulteration and food safety, social security and social insurance and benefits come under the concurrent list, where both the Union government and the states have joint responsibility.

Should Health Remain a State Subject?

Over the years, a strong case has often been made for bringing all of health into the concurrent list. The main argument advanced in favour of this shift is that the Centre has far more resources to ensure universal health care. Others have argued that this would enable Parliament to enact a Right to Health legislation, which it currently cannot do since health is a state subject. Moreover, Central intervention is essential to ensure that as a nation we meet our obligations under a number of international treaties. A third argument frequently raised is that many states do not have the capacity to plan and manage their state health system. And finally, that political will can be limited in many states, especially states with poor outcomes.

However, given the diversity and complexity of health-care provisions and the evolution of health systems over time, there are stronger arguments against shifting it out of the state list. States have wide differences in social determinants, levels of health systems development, institutional capacity and political will. Rather than assuming that a Central authority can impose uniform processes, standards and outcomes, a federal structure and state autonomy in health planning and financing is vital if we are to have a chance at accountable delivery on the ground. While the point about low state capacity is valid, the solution is to build the necessary capacity in states. States like Kerala and Tamil Nadu developed better health systems not because of Central guidance, but because they invested in building better capacity to plan and implement. In any case, centralization has posed problems even in the current federal architecture; bringing health care into the concurrent list would only signal further centralization in a counterproductive direction.

A major reason for excessive centralization has been lack of fiscal space within states to invest in health systems, especially since the nineties. When more health funding does flow in from the Centre, it comes in the form of specific Centrally Sponsored Schemes (CSS), with relatively inflexible designs. External donors have also funded many CSSs, and agreements with them have further contributed to such inflexibility. Thus, a situation has evolved where the health workforce and infrastructure is paid for by the state, accounting for 70 to 90 per cent of total public health expenditure, while the remaining 10 to 30 per cent that the Centre provides actually determines health programmes.

Experience with the National Health Mission

In recent times, the National Health Mission (NHM), which began initially as the National Rural Health Mission, broke with this logic and started funding the strengthening of state health systems. This was justified as a supplement to Central funding of the main vertical programmes, primarily Reproductive and Child Health (RCH), and the control of tuberculosis, vector-borne diseases, HIV and leprosy. A belated recognition that the Centrally sponsored vertical programmes could not succeed in the absence of state health systems strengthening and that Central support was required for such strengthening justified this approach.

Towards this end, district health planning was insisted upon and these district health plans were aggregated into a state health plan that was to be sanctioned and funded by joint mechanisms, with the Centre providing over 80 per cent of the funds. Such district plans had the potential to address a larger range of health care needs through better public health infrastructure and human resources. However, by 2010, there was a strong reversal within NHM, with a return to an emphasis on vertical programmes and a very selective package of services with a tightly controlled budget. States were unhappy with this development and felt this was excessive centralization, even though when compared to other vertical programmes, the NHM still had greater flexibility. On the other hand, rigidities of the financing process, which limited discretionary fund allocation at the state and district levels, were a response intended to prevent leakage. In 2009, major media coverage of corruption and crime reported from Uttar Pradesh related to NHM funds had made the Centre wary of extending flexibility in using financial resources.[1]

Recent Centralization Trends

In contrast to the struggles to design the NHM in a way that strikes a better balance of powers between Centre and the states, the Rashtriya Swasthya Bima Yojana (RSBY), launched in 2008, was designed as a Central programme, where states only had the option to join in. Many did not, and started their own government-funded health insurance programmes. In 2018, the Pradhan Mantri Jan Arogya Yojana (PMJAY) was launched as a Central programme. Not all states were keen on giving up their programmes to join this new scheme, but the pressure was to incorporate all of them, and over time, only a few states could hold out.[2] There had clearly been a shift.

The old debate around federalism in Center–state relationships had taken place in a context where the government was the main provider of services and scheme design, and budgetary allocations were made for this purpose. But by 2018, not only had private players become major providers, but policy direction was also explicitly directed towards expanding the role of the private sector in the provision of health-care services and limiting government role to a purchaser of services. Centralization was now about regulations and regulatory frameworks, about encouraging private provisioning of services on a pan-India basis through a centralized all-India publicly funded health insurance model operating on a centralized digital platform governed by the NHA. Both the corporate health-care industry and the Central government sought increased Central authority to enable this.

The National Health Agency was set up in May 2018 to manage the PMJAY, overseen by the NITI Aayog. The agency was created by a cabinet decision, and by a similar decision renamed as National Health Authority in January 2019. Its mandate has since extended to leading efforts to scale up public–private partnerships where it works directly with the states as well. In 2020, the NHA was designated as the nodal agency for implementing India's Digital Health Mission (NDHM). In this regard, the NHA is unlike other authorities, like the Telecom Regulatory Authority, which have been created by an act of Parliament and do not overlap with the service delivery of central ministries and their departments.

Besides overseeing the PMJAY and the NDHM, the NHA mandate is also to facilitate outsourcing of public hospitals currently managed by state departments of health, so as to shift the role of government from provider to purchaser of health-care services. Thus, in this new context, the call to bring health into the concurrent list becomes an enabler for privatization of health care. If purchase through market-based insurance schemes and purchasing care from corporate-owned 'integrated health care providers' gains acceptance as the main approach to providing free services, bringing all of health care under the concurrent list and even the right to health bill could become the vehicle to increase public financing of the private sector for service delivery. This is a route that has been followed by many countries. But has this led towards universal health coverage? In practice, because of financial constraints, the package of essential services and beneficiaries are far from universal. They remain selective. Instead, it is an unregulated private market in health care which seems to grow in this space, and this market is characterized by considerable inequities in access, financial protection and outcomes.

Coordination and Mutual Accountability

What is the way forward? In the interests of democratic, federal governance that is responsive to health-care needs and equity in health care, there is a greater case for strengthening the role of health and health care as the state's prerogative, with the Centre providing the technical and financial support required. Good governance means that we need to work out ways by which the Union government and state governments are held mutually accountable to act in a coordinated manner to make policies and implement strategies that lead towards the realization of health and health care as a right, substantively and not just legislatively. This requires redesigning institutional arrangements and the current fiscal architecture and systems.

The trend so far has been that the Union government has seen itself as responsible only for Centrally Sponsored Schemes and not for state health systems strengthening. This changed in a very limited way with the National Health Mission, but not to the extent that the Centre saw itself as being responsible for the realization of the right to health in the states. When it came to that, despite the decreasing fiscal space that states had, the responsibility was seen as that of the states.

This division of work between the Centre and states changes when it comes to dealing with the private sector. Now the major concern is not budgetary allocation, systems strengthening and implementation, but defining policy with regard to the stewardship role of the government. Currently, the Union government's priorities include: a) promotion of profitability in private markets for medical and health professional education, in innovation and manufacture of medical products, and in promotion of health care as an industry; b) the attraction of foreign direct investment in the health sector; c) the regulation of professional education and professional practice; and d) mechanisms of contracting out public infrastructure and contracting in private providers for expanding public services. This has led to high degrees of centralization, with reduced powers not only to state governments but also to the Union Ministry of Health and Family Welfare and the creation of new institutional structures like the National Health Authority, the National Digital Health Mission and the National Medical Commission. Much of this centralization is justified on the basis of the Centre having the institutional capacity to manage these functions, and states being unable to do so.

In such a distribution of resources and powers between the Centre and the states, it becomes unclear as to who has the primary accountability for health outcomes and health rights. The COVID-19 pandemic and government response highlight this problem and its consequences. All public health measures and the vast majority of curative health care that were required were provided by the public sector, with the private sector, even when it was contracted in, having a very marginal role. The budget-financed public sector was held accountable for this by the media and even by courts. The case of the vaccine policy, in particular, has brought multiple issues in terms of production, regulation, procurement and distribution across the public and private sector and the Centre and the states to the fore. The 2021 suo motu Supreme Court hearings on this matter are becoming an important judicial effort to define the Centre's and states' mutual accountability to the realization of specific health rights and may provide some interesting insights going forward.

Beyond the legal and accountability framework, the states and the Union government also require the institutional capacity for both health systems delivery and the increasingly vital role of stewardship of the health sector. The so-called lack of such capacity in the states is often an important justification for further centralization. We would argue, however, that there is lack of public health management capacity to deliver universal health care and health rights both at the Centre and the states. In the next section we outline some of the reasons for this deficit and some of the key approaches required for building institutional capacity for health in India.

Institutional Capacity in Health Governance: An Evolving and Abiding Antagonism

Health administration as we see it today, is in part, a legacy of British colonial rule. The distribution of the functions of health governance into what is known today as union, concurrent and state lists of the Constitution began in 1935. The first public health institutions were also created under the British, the first of which was the Central Research Institute (CRI) at Kasauli in 1905, from which later emerged the Indian Council for Medical Research, which much more recently also evolved into the Department of Health Research. The CRI Kasauli continues with a more focused mandate around production and certification of a few vaccines. The National Institute for Communicable Disease (which is now renamed the National Centre for Disease Control), the All India Institute of Public Health and Hygiene, as well as another eight national institutions began from an early twentieth-century pre-Independence initiative. Medical professionals managed the senior administration of hospitals, while commissioners of public health headed research institutions.

With Independence, the posts of Director General, Indian Medical Services and Public Health (PH) Commissioner were integrated in the post of DGHS, both at the Centre and in the states. The Office of the Directorate General of Health Services now represented the technical wing. As distinct from the directorate, there was a Department of Health staffed by general administrators of the Indian Administrative Service.

Until the early eighties, the Office of the Directorate was the main strength of the Central health ministry with about fifty-five officers, whereas there were only seven or eight officers in the Department of Health, and its position in the states was similar. From the early eighties, the strength of general administrators rose considerably and the role of the office of the DGHS weakened. In the nineties, following an agitation by the Central Health Services doctors, a commission was constituted. Its report, called the Tikkoo Commission Report, presented a set of recommendations that assured promotion and much better terms of service for the Central Health Services. However, it failed to engage with the question of how best to assure adequate capacity in its leadership and consider the architecture of governance that was required in practice. There were no processes put in place either to select officers or build capacity for administrative or policy positions. For instance, many officers were promoted only towards the end of their service period and moved directly from clinical work or hospital administration into senior administrative positions requiring knowledge of policy and systems. Public health experience or knowledge was not mandatory. The Central Health Services had close to 4612 officers, of whom about 104 were in the public health cadre.[3] This was the context in which the importance of general administrators in decision-making increased greatly.

Much of the discussion on institutional capacity in health governance becomes tied to the division of powers between the technical wing—the Directorates of Health—and the administrative wing—the Departments of Health. Numerous reports on improving governance focus on the reporting relationships and distribution of powers, characterized by drawing and re-drawing organograms expressing these relationships. This is true both in the states and in the Central ministries of health and medical education. IAS officers in the departments bemoan the lack of technical capacity in the directorates. The directorates attribute poor performance to uninformed dominance by the general administrator over the technical wings.

In the course of work and numerous reform discussions involving the Directorate of Health Services, the frustrations within the Directorate were frequently expressed. This included the criticisms that bureaucrats and contractual advisers, with little experience in public health, have not only increasingly assumed these responsibilities and head technical divisions, but also that non-health bodies such as the erstwhile Planning Commission and Ministry of Expenditure exercised decision-making on technical matters related to health. From the point of view of the DGHS, this represented a serious shrinking of space and scope for technical decision-making.

In this context, the rise and growth of the governance structures of the National Health Mission drew particular resistance. Though the Director General's office was substantially represented and consulted, in practice, decision-making was largely shifted to the IAS cadre. To the general administrator, this was a consequence of the loss of capacity in the technical cadre, who could not rise to the occasion, but the technical cadre did not see it that way.

Many new institutions like the National Health Systems Resource Centre and State Health Resource Centres have also been set up to fill these gaps, but few sustain as dynamic bodies. And in the states, as general administrators are subject to frequent transfers, and political pressures on key appointments are persistent, the problems of institutional capacity are often exacerbated. What are the reasons for the inability to build the necessary professional and managerial capacity in the departments, in the directorates and in the public health institutions, both at the Centre and in the state? And what can be done about this? We look at two critical aspects below and the principles and possibilities available to us for doing things differently.

Organizational Structure, Design and Human Resources

All directorates are made up of officers whose posts are organized as an administrative hierarchy. They consist of the director-general, the additional director-general, then joint directors, deputy director commissioner, assistant commissioner, chief medical officers and so on. The general administrators are also organized along such a hierarchy: secretary, additional secretary, joint secretary, deputy secretary, directors, and so on. These positions are secured by promotion, and promotion is largely on basis of seniority. To fulfil their work there is a clerical team of a section officer and clerical staff under them. There is no provision for them to have a multi-level, technically skilled staff with the right mix of skills. Thus, a deputy commissioner in charge of an immunization programme would have to share a section officer and three or four clerical staff who would take care of issuing orders and maintaining files of orders issued and correspondence related to this. What she may really need is a young expert in logistics, another with an immunology background, a third with health communication skills and perhaps another junior medical person to help in field visits. But no government structure allows for such positions. Instead, it is designed purely to perform an administrative function suitable for allocation of power and resources, but unable to assess and use scientific information relevant to decision-making and implementation.

Further, most of the directorate medical officers have clinical qualifications and experience but very few have any public health knowledge or experience before they join their administrative post. Very few states have a public health cadre for this purpose.

The only exceptions are Tamil Nadu and, to some extent, Odisha and Maharashtra. Tamil Nadu also has a provision that a joint director of the public health cadre can interchangeably work as a professor of preventive and social medicine in a medical college with opportunities to gain teaching and research experience in an area. Faculty of medical colleges can also work in administration at state and district level. But no other state has this provision. At the Centre, as mentioned earlier, across a 3000-person strong central health services, less than a 100 have public health qualifications. Many therefore have little awareness of public health as a science and public health management as specific domain of knowledge and practice.

They could alternatively learn on the job but quite often the career path defined for them does not give them the necessary experience to do so. Many have been working in dispensaries and hospitals before suddenly assuming charge of a national programme. A general administrator of the IAS cadre works for some time as a sub-district or block officer, then for a considerable degree of time as a district magistrate and then in various positions in state departments before handling senior positions at the national level. But most technical officers at the national level have almost no district or state experience. There are few, if any, opportunities for gathering different but essential experiences.

IAS officers are often allowed to work with civil society organizations, with private sector organizations and with international organizations to have different types of exposure and develop different skills. None of these would generally be permissible to any technical officer. Opportunities to develop management skills and enhance knowledge of public health science are limited to occasional training programmes. This is far from sufficient.

To overcome these barriers, the main reform measures that have been suggested aim at a) developing a public health management cadre who work at mid-level management positions and have exposure to policy work before they are posted in senior administrative positions; b) allowing lateral entry of suitable skills and c) building new institutional structures that can recruit and nurture specific management skills required. A more radical revision of service rules could also be thought of.

Developing a Public-Health Cadre. The first and the most often cited reform is the creation of a public health cadre. Despite decades of promotion of this as the solution, only three or four states have implemented the approach. In the state of Tamil Nadu, after a few years of service, medical officers are allowed to opt out of the general cadre into a smaller public health cadre. These officers are freed from clinical work, qualify for a non-practising allowance, and are then required to obtain a formal public health qualification, diploma or degree. They are posted as administrators at sub-district and district level and rise faster to senior positions. They have a better grasp of health policy and health systems and public health and their positions are interchangeable with that of the faculty of preventive medicine and public health in the government medical colleges. A number of sources have attributed Tamil Nadu health systems performance to the existence of this cadre.[4] However, even these officers struggle at higher levels of policy and systems work. Deputations to international organizations or even civil society organizations or academic exposure to public policy could help further develop these skills.

Contractual Consultants. A less effective approach that has been adopted is to hire technical officers on a contractual basis to assist the regular officer in such work. These are usually one-year contracts with no assurance of renewal, and the salaries and benefits are typically lower than for regular employees. Very often, departments have to get an external aid partner to do the hiring and place the consultant at their disposal. Alternatively, arrangements are made for hiring such consultants in one of the Centrally sponsored programmes like the NHM, the disease control programmes, or in one of the autonomous para-statal bodies like NHSRC, who do the hiring on their behalf. As a gap-filling ad hoc arrangement this often works, but in the long term, the institutional capacity does not stabilize or grow as there is high turnover and little capacity building possible in contractual staff. There is a need to create regular positions for persons with these interdisciplinary public health-related skills and to allow them to grow within the system with the necessary job security and support.

New Institutional Structures: The Para-statal Bodies. The third approach is the emergence of new institutional structures, often referred to as para-statal bodies. These are not formally within the government and therefore at least some of the workforce rules do not apply and enable more flexible hiring of staff, the creation of necessary teams and the organization of work processes. Yet in other ways their functioning retains many elements of governmental organizational systems and cultures. There are a significant number of such new institutional forms that have emerged in recent years, including the state and district health societies of the NHM, as well as statutory regulatory bodies like the Food Safety and Standards Authority of India (FFSAI) and the Central Drugs and Standards Control Organization (CDSCO), the trusts created to manage the government-funded public insurance programmes, the state medical service corporations for procurement and logistics, and new institutions created for training and research. Unfortunately, not all of these have done well and most are poorly integrated into governance functions. Positive examples of successful institutions need to be identified and studied to understand the possibilities by which the required institutional capacity can be created.

The Ecosystem of Knowledge and Research Institutions

Health is a scientific and knowledge-intensive field of practice, and the capacity to govern lies not only within the ministry but, just as importantly, within several research and knowledge management institutions associated with it. Those under the Department of Health and Family Welfare can be categorized into three main groups. In the first are six institutions directly concerned with pharmaceuticals, biologicals and vaccines. In the second are research institutions with contribution to disease control and public health and the third are three institutions that come directly under the ministry for policy, research and capacity building.

Table 1: Knowledge Management/Technical Institutions under the Department of Health and Family Welfare

For Pharmaceuticals and Biologicals	For Disease Prevention and Public Health	For Policy, Research and Capacity Building
Indian Pharmacopia Commission	National Centre for Disease Control (NCDC)	National Institute of Health and Family Welfare (NIHFW)
The National Institute of Biologicals (Noida)	National Tuberculosis Institute, (NTI), Bengaluru	International Institute of Population Sciences (IIPS)
Institute of Serology, Kolkata	Central Leprosy Training & Research Institution, (CLTRI) Chengalpattu	The National Health Systems Resource Centre (NHSRC)
BCG Vaccine Lab, Chennai	All India Institute of Hygiene & Public Health	
Central Research Institute, Kasauli	The Central Bureau of Health Intelligence	
Pasteur Institute of India, Coonoor	The Central Health Education Bureau	

All the institutions in the first two columns are governed directly by the Office of the Director General of Health Services, through a senior cadre officer posted as the director. They do not have any formal autonomy.

The Indian Pharmacopia Commission and the National Institute of Biologicals define the standards for Indian drugs and biologicals and play an important role not only in regulation, but also in fostering indigenous manufacturing. The remaining four institutions in the group are almost a century old and were once the leading research and manufacturing units for medical technologies in the developing world.

This is also true for many of the institutions in the second column, which are more explicitly research and capacity building institutions for disease control. The NCDC is a relatively dynamic institution, playing a major role in programme management and in disease surveillance. Meant to be the Indian equivalent of the Centers for Disease Control (CDC), USA, it, however, has nowhere near the same prestige or capacity for setting policy in technical areas. When the COVID-19 pandemic broke out, it should have been in the lead but was not. The last three institutions in this category have a very limited presence in national policy or strategy implementation, though each of these have a long history.

The institutions in the third column have a policy and research function, and also undertake extensive public health capacity building. Most states have similar state-level institutions. They have a fair degree of autonomy, with a governing board chaired by the Health Minister or Secretary. The institutions above have been mentioned in some detail to underline the fact that India has built up a tremendous institutional base in the area of public health-relevant research. Many of these institutions have had their moments of glory, and some have been leading international institutions. Unfortunately, over time, their contributions have become much more limited, and a few are almost non-functional.

Under the Department of Health Research within the same ministry, there are thirty national research institutions, many of which have a good track record of work in their specialized area. There are also research institutions under Department of Biotechnology and the Department of Science and Technology that have the potential to contribute to the making of Indian health policies and strategies in their domains. The problems they face are not dissimilar to the problems that we listed for the lack of institutional capacity in the directorate and departments of health. Many of these research institutions do not have the necessary legal and functional autonomy. Even where they have the legal autonomy, a mass of inappropriate government rules relating to recruitment, terms of service, programme management, research funding etc. come in the way. Internal capacity building is limited and sporadic. And there is limited permeability between these organizations and the larger body of academic work in health policy and health systems research.

As a result of the poor capacity of these institutions, the government resorts to a high level of dependence on external aid agencies for technical assistance and, increasingly, on corporate consultancy firms. There are serious conflicts of interest and sovereignty issues in such deepening dependence.

Revitalizing Public Health Research Institutions

Turning around these institutions is not easy, but this is our central challenge. The starting point for the revitalization and strengthening of our public research institutions is, of course, much greater financial and administrative autonomy. This in turn requires a governing board with the skills and perspective to provide leadership to their development. Internally, there is a need to build up an administrative culture that is far more participatory, with decentralization of functions as required. Leadership must come from the technical officers, not the general administrators. But there must be a clear process of grooming the leadership in administrative and policy work, with sufficient national and international exposure before individuals are chosen from within for the top post. This is essential to ensuring that there are people with vision, experience and credibility at the helm, and a work culture with professional pride at all levels. In the area of knowledge management, well-chosen knowledge partnerships with benchmarked national and international institutions should also be carefully crafted and put in place.

All of these are considered 'technical' aspects of governance, but they do not exist apart from the larger policy environment. The repeated ideological stereotyping of the public institution as something that is inherently inefficient and bound to fail, and a glorification of commercial institutions as designed for success are caricatures both in India and abroad. In most developed nations, public institutions and public financing has been the key to building up robust health systems and health research institutions. Moreover, even for the private health-care sector to be viable and sustainable, well-functioning public institutions of governance and research are required.

The confidence and skills for a much better quality of public health administration have to be re-learnt.

Authors' Note

The materials and analysis presented in the essay draw in large measure on work conducted by T. Sundararaman during his tenure as Executive Director of the National Health Systems Resource Centre and service on multiple committees and commissions set up to examine the critical challenges of health systems governance and reform. Much of this information, however, remains formally unpublished or undocumented. The essay also draws on the knowledge and insights generously shared in the course of discussions with a wide range of experts, activists and administrators who have served in different public health institutions in India. All errors are our own.

Innovations for Health Systems Strengthening in Chhattisgarh: A Public–Community Partnership

T.S. Singh Deo

Chhattisgarh is a relatively young Indian state, formed in the year 2000. It now has 28 districts with around 28 million persons, 77 per cent of the population living in rural areas. Scheduled tribes constitute 31 per cent of Chhattisgarh's population—almost four times the national average of 8 per cent—but remain its most vulnerable section. The tribal districts face multiple challenges in delivering health care and other services due to difficult geography, poor infrastructure and high levels of poverty. Chhattisgarh is one of the poorest states in India in terms of proportion of population living below the poverty line. The areas inhabited by tribal population were relatively outside the mainstream of the state and civil society, living in harmony with nature's abundance. However, as other parts of the state developed, there was exploitation of natural resources and the tribals and farmers were left impoverished, their way of life disrupted and malnutrition becoming rampant. The state is now proactive in making efforts to improve its people's health and wellbeing.

The state currently faces a double burden of the COVID-19 pandemic and the continuing historical challenges. This essay brings some insight into the experiments and innovations in governance systems that address historical injustices and modernize, yet without giving up the traditional wisdom and knowledge, to build a robust health system for a healthy Chhattisgarh.

The Case for Universal Health Care in Chhattisgarh

Out-of-pocket medical expenses make up about 62 per cent of all health-care costs in India. As Insurance Regulatory & Development Authority of India (IRDAI) Chairman T.S. Vijayan notes, 'This is extremely high and leads to impoverishment of patients. In comparison, out of pocket hospital expenses in developed countries such as the U.S. and the U.K. are 20 per cent and about 20–25 per cent in BRICS countries.'[1]

Table 1: Out-of-Pocket Expenditure on Health care in Chhattisgarh and All India

INDICATORS	CHHATTISGARH		ALL INDIA	
	Rural	*Urban*	*Rural*	*Urban*
OUT-OF-POCKET EXPENDITURES ON HEALTH CARE (OOPE)				
Hospitalization Expenditure (excluding child birth)				
OOPE per hospitalized case—All	₹11,957	₹21,711	₹14,473	₹21,985
OOPE per hospitalized case—Public	₹3801	₹3172	₹5369	₹7189
OOPE per hospitalized case—Private	₹19,928	₹29,445	₹21,034	₹28,958
Childbirth Expenditure (as inpatient) (In Rs.)				
OOPE per childbirth—All	₹2919	₹7895	₹5518	₹11,033
OOPE per childbirth—Public	₹1409	₹3300	₹1572	₹2094

OOPE per childbirth— Private	₹10,675	₹15,845	₹14,727	₹19,107
NON-HOSPITALIZED EXPENDITURE AS A PROPORTION OF OUTPATIENT MEDICAL EXPENDITURE				
Diagnostics Expenditure	**4 per cent**	**6 per cent**	11 per cent	12 per cent
Drugs Expenditure— Private	**83 per cent**	**83 per cent**	73 per cent	68 per cent
Drugs Expenditure—Public	**92 per cent**	**93 per cent**	76 per cent	67 per cent
HOSPITALIZATION EXPENDITURE (RS.)				
Average expenditure (medical & non-medical) per hospitalized case—All	₹5433	₹4655	₹7724	₹13,690
Average medical expenditure per hospitalized case—All	₹5003	₹4317	₹6682	₹12,456
CATASTROPHIC HOUSEHOLDS (Household's OOPE > 10 per cent of Total Household Consumption Expenditure)				
Households reporting catastrophic OOPE	**16 per cent**		**15 per cent**	

* **Household Health-Care Utilization & Expenditure in India: State Fact Sheets, Health-Care Financing Division, National Health Systems Resource Centre, Ministry of Health and Family Welfare, Government of India (2014)**

Ensuring that all people remain or become healthy by obtaining the health services they need without suffering financial hardship is a societal responsibility. This requires ensuring equitable access for all Indian citizens, resident in any part of the country, regardless of the income level, social status, gender, caste or religion, to Affordable, Accountable, Appropriate Health Services of Assured Quality (promotive, preventive, curative and rehabilitative) as well as public health services addressing the wider determinants of health delivered to individuals and populations, with the government being the guarantor and enabler, although not necessarily the provider of health and related services.

It is important to also take note of the dual role of health care in directly making our lives better—it reduces impoverishment in ways that matter to all human beings and helps to remove poverty, assessed even in purely economic terms. Health care plays a role in reducing economic poverty partly due to the greater productivity of a healthy population, leading to higher wages and larger rewards from more effective work, but also because Universal Health Coverage (UHC) makes it less likely that vulnerable, uninsured people would be made destitute by medical expenses far beyond their means.

The mutual support that health care and economic development can provide has been brought out extensively by the results of UHC-oriented policies in Asia, from Japan to Singapore. The complementary nature of health advancement and economic progress is also illustrated in the comparative experiences of different states within India. Despite its poverty, Kerala did manage to run an effective UHC programme that has contributed greatly to its having, by some margin, the longest life expectancy in India and the lowest rates of infant and child mortality, among its other health accomplishments. But in addition to 'social achievements', Kerala has also grown faster in purely economic terms. After all, there are no influences as strong in raising the productivity of labour as health, education and skill formation—a foundational connection to which Adam Smith gave much attention. In fact, the previously poor state of Kerala, thanks to its universal health care and universal schooling now has the highest per capita income among all the states in India. Tamil Nadu and Himachal Pradesh, both of which have made substantial moves towards the provision of education and basic health care for all, too have progressed admirably and now belong solidly among the richer Indian states.

Achieving UHC requires three sets of inputs:

- **Social Demand** from the people for universal health care for all illnesses at a place convenient to all.

- **Political Commitment** to deliver UHC. This will require legislation for Right to Health.
- **Knowledge of the Processes** to implement the elements of UHC, which includes setting up appropriate institutions to govern, implement and monitor UHC, financial management, setting up appropriate human resources, ensuring supplies of resources such as drugs, diagnostics and equipment and community-based monitoring.

As has been analysed by many economists, most notably Kenneth Arrow, there cannot be a well-informed competitive market equilibrium in the field of medical attention and delivery of medical services because of what economists call 'Asymmetric Information'. Patients do not typically know what treatment they need for their ailments, or what medicine would work, or even what exactly the doctor is giving to them as a remedy, and this vitiates the efficiency of market competition. This applies to the market for health insurance as well, since insurance companies cannot fully know what patients' health conditions are. This makes markets for private health insurance inescapably inefficient, even in terms of the narrow logic of market allocation. And there is, in addition, the much bigger problem—private insurance companies, if unrestrained by regulations, have a strong financial interest in excluding patients who are taken to be 'high-risk'. As a result, in the absence of a well-organized public health system covering all, many patients remain vulnerable to exploitation.

Therefore, UHC is achievable only through tax-based financing, and for which a minimum of 2.5 per cent of GDP is needed.[2] It must be delivered primarily through a strengthened public health system that will provide comprehensive primary, secondary and tertiary health care to all. It also will act as a benchmark for the private sector, whose services will have to be creatively in-sourced where needed.

UHC would require increased resources, even though good governance can lead to major cost savings over time. The initial years would require investment in upgrading as well as building infrastructure. In Chhattisgarh, an investment of Rs 7100 crore is needed annually to deliver Universal Health Care to all 3.14 crore residents.[3]

Key to ensuring Universal Health Care would be a Right to Health Care Act to establish an autonomous authority to look into administrative, financial and regulatory frameworks for the health-care systems and establish rights, duties and liabilities of health-care receivers and providers. The Public Health Care System should be truly for the people of Chhattisgarh and not just the poor.

'A service just for the Poor will end up becoming a Poor Service'[4]

Situational Analysis

At the time of its formation, Chhattisgarh inherited a very weak health-care system. It performed poorly in key health indicators, with Infant Mortality Rate being seventy-nine per 1000 live births (when the all-India IMR was sixty-six), high malnutrition rates and low rates of access to safe drinking water and use of sanitary toilets. The state had only one medical college, nine district hospitals, and a network of too few rural health centres that were mostly lacking in basic infrastructure and human resource for any functionality. Media outreach was extremely low, heightening the lack of health education in these areas.

Over the years, the state focused on increasing the government health-care infrastructure and its functionality so as to reach the poor and the marginalized. Currently, the state has around 5200 Sub-Health Centres (SHCs), 796 Primary Health Centres (PHCs), 170 Community Health Centres (CHCs), twenty-six District Hospitals and six Medical Colleges.[5] A key constraint faced by the state was the inadequate availability of qualified medical professionals. However, over the last two decades, Chhattisgarh has outperformed many other states in important areas of health and health care. When a comparison was made among the states in terms of quantum of change achieved in key indicators from the National Family Health Survey-Round 2 (NFHS-2) to NFHS-3 (1998–99 to 2005–06), Chhattisgarh achieved first position. A decade later, when the index was applied for change between NFHS-3 and NFHS-4 (2005–06 to 2015–16), Chhattisgarh stood first again.

The following table on some key health indicators reported by the National Family Health Survey (NFHS) rounds 2, 3 and 4 shows the state's achievements in implementation and outcomes.

Table 2: Key Progress Indicators in Health

Indicators	NFHS-2 (1998–1999)	NFHS-3 (2005–06)	NFHS-4 (2015–2016)	NFHS – 5 (2019-21)
Infant mortality rate (IMR)	80.9	71	54	44.3
Under-five mortality rate (U5MR)	122.7	90	64	50.4
Households with an improved drinking-water source (per cent)	37.6	77.9	91.1	95.5
Households using improved sanitation facility (per cent)	13.5	14.6	32.7	76.8
Households using iodized salt (per cent)	60.4	79.0	99.1	98.5
Institutional births (per cent)	13.8	15.7	70.2	85.7

Children aged under five years whose birth was registered (per cent)	NA	73.0	86.1	96.6
Children aged 12–23 months fully immunized (BCG, measles, and three doses each of polio and DPT) (per cent)	21.8	48.7	76.4	79.7

Source: National Family Health Survey, India

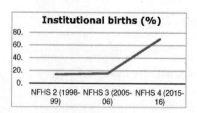

Graph 1: Trends in Percentage Institutional Deliveries in Chhattisgarh

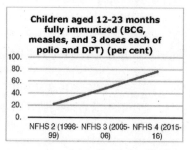

Graph 2: Trends in Percentage of Fully Immunized Children in Chhattisgarh

Infant mortality rate decreased from 80.9 per cent (1998–99) to 71 per cent (2005–06) to 54 per cent (2015–16), suggesting increasing access to better health care for mothers during pregnancy in these past years, including access to antenatal check-ups, vaccines and iron and folic acid supplementation. Graph 1 depicts the increase in institutional deliveries. Under-five mortality rate too has decreased by almost half from 122.7 per cent (2005–06) to 64 per cent (2015–16). Graph 2 depicts the percentage of children aged 12–23 months who are fully immunized with the required doses of BCG, measles and polio and DPT, as reported in NFHS rounds 2, 3 and 4. It illustrates a steady increase in the figures over the years, implying a healthy future for children from Chhattisgarh.

SOME KEY POLICY CHANGES THAT TRANSFORMED THE NARRATIVE

With a policy steadfastness, the new Chhattisgarh is now a model of evolving health systems. The government initiatives are exemplary efforts to enhance the health-care ecosystem into a robust one. Policies designed around community-centric mechanisms and grievance redressal have brought a swift change in the health narrative of the state. The decision of the government to make treatment methods more inclusive also shows its enthusiasm towards its culturally rich history and traditions.

Swimming Against the Tide: Focus on Public System Strengthening Instead of a Private Sector-Led Insurance Model

Chhattisgarh, like the rest of the country, has a mixed health-care system with public and private providers. The first set of improvements was directed at community-level government services in the coverage of child immunization and antenatal care, with a somewhat longer effort to achieve desired improvements in disease-control. The most difficult area to improve in Chhattisgarh, however, was the availability and quality of institutional care. The state inherited poor infrastructure and a very poor availability of doctors, nurses and other medical human resources.

Chhattisgarh initially experimented with developing its hospital services through an insurance model. It was a leading implementer of the Rashtriya Swasthya Bima Yojana (RSBY) or the National Health Insurance Scheme for below-poverty-line (BPL) families from 2008 onwards. It added its own insurance schemes to increase coverage of insurance to around 80 per cent of the population. The vertical cover was increased manifold in 2018 when the state adopted the new national scheme of PMJAY. The Pradhan Mantri Jan Arogya Yojana (PMJAY) under the Ayushman Bharat scheme, the upscaled version of the hitherto implemented health insurance programme called Rashtriya Swasthya Bima Yojana (RSBY), is a health insurance scheme where the Central government pays a premium to the insurance company, which guarantees health care only for certain illnesses for those who are admitted to empanelled hospitals for selected people judged to be poor by the SECC survey of 2011, and up to an amount of Rs 5,00,000 per family. To be noted is that the premium given by the Central government covers only up to Rs 50,000 per family and any additional expenses is paid by the state government via a trust model (for the state of Chhattisgarh).

However, various studies showed that the coverage provided though such schemes had several important gaps.[6] The schemes tried to improve access to health care by empanelling private hospitals. However, most of the private sector was concentrated in a few urban areas. The neediest populations lived in rural areas, including the tribal belts, where the availability of services did not increase despite people getting enrolled under insurance programmes. PMJAY does not look after those illnesses that require outpatient care and does not look at preventive or promotive health care. Primary and secondary care account for 70 per cent of all health-care interventions.

Further, the out-of-pocket expenditure for those able to utilize the insurance schemes did not come down. Private hospitals continued to charge extra from majority of patients and it was difficult to regulate and control such practices. Patients going in for simple illnesses ended up being subjected to unnecessary procedures by private hospitals, highlighted by instances such as where patients had their uteruses removed without due medical process.[2] There was a mushrooming of private facilities, and insurance schemes helped the migration of financial and human resources from the public to private sector. Private health-care practitioners provide a narrow and selective range of services and cater to the needs of the richer population to gain profits.

The idea that it might be more desirable to invest in and strengthen the government sector was akin to swimming against the tide because of the wider belief of policymakers that people *preferred* private services to public health care, which was perceived as non-responsive and of poor quality. Further, the predominant perception was that the private sector provided close to 80 per cent of the medical care in India and, therefore, any approach without aid from this sector or which did not rely on it was bound to fail. Chhattisgarh, however, took the bold decision to build its public sector both for primary and ambulatory care as well as for inpatient hospital care.

Prior to 2019, the Hybrid Health Financing Model was adopted by the Ayushman Bharat Scheme, where a private insurance company was tendered. The Ayushman Bharat Scheme would provide a maximum sum of Rs 1102 per family, which was shared between the Centre and state in the ratio of 60:40. When a tender was done for an insurance company to provide a health coverage using this money, the lowest bidder bid Rs 1100 per family and provided for only Rs 50,000 coverage (sum insured) for the family. Thus, if the family incurred a health claim of, say, Rs 1,00,000, the amount provided by Ayushman Bharat would cover only Rs 50,000 and the state government would have to pay the additional Rs 50,000 from its treasury. This was settled internally by the State Nodal Agency. Thus, the claim that Ayushman Bharat provided for a coverage of Rs 5 lakh per family is not completely accurate.

Even this allocation was available for only 63 per cent (42 lakh) families as per the SECC database. The remaining families (excluding the families of government servants who accounted for around 6 per cent) were provided a coverage of Rs 50,000 only under the Mukhyamantri Swasthya Bima Yojana (MSBY).

In 2019, it was then decided by the Chhattisgarh government to merge all existing Health Coverage Schemes (AB, MVSSY, Sanjeevni, Bal Shravan Yojna, Bal Hriday Yojna, Chirayu, etc.) into the Ayushman Bharat–Dr. Khubchand Baghel Swasth Sahayata Yojna, which would provide a coverage of Rs 5 lakh for all families with Antyodaya Ration Cards (90 per cent of families in Chhattisgarh) and the remaining families (excluding the families of government servants) would be provided a coverage of Rs 50,000 only.[7] Apart from this, under the Mukhyamantri Vishesh Swasth Sahayata Yojna, a support of up to Rs 20 lakh was to be provided for fourteen rare conditions for all families of Chhattisgarh (families above the poverty line would need the approval of the chief minister).

It was also decided to shift from the Hybrid Health Financing Model, which had a very high administrative expense (15 per cent), to the Trust Health Financing Model. Under the Trust Model, it was decided to use the services of two Third Party Administrators. One TPA would be responsible for claim processing and the second TPA would audit the claims processed by the first TPA. By deviating from the national model, the state is thus saving large sums in premiums by directly handling the insurance operations rather than through a private company.

The Trust Model has shifted the emphasis from empanelling the private sector to a more judicious mix of public and private providers, building on the strengths of each. The funding imbalance between private and public sector has been corrected to an extent, from only 15 per cent of the claim amount going to the public sector till 2018, to around 45 per cent of the claim amount going to it in 2021. With a clear goal of strengthening the public system, incentives for HR in public hospitals have been enhanced.

Comprehensive Urban Health Programme

The approach to addressing urban health must differ from that taken for rural health care. The urban setting's high population density coupled with sanitation and pollution issues make it paramount to have a robust and accessible primary, preventive and palliative health-care system with a strong community outreach component to address the social determinants of health.[8]

A two-tier primary urban health infrastructure is proposed in the state:

- Hamar Clinics
- Hamar Aspataal

A. Hamar Clinic

The principle of Hamar Clinic (Urban Health and Wellness Centres) locations is that they become the first port of call for individuals and families in urban areas and should cater to a population of 10,000–15,000 persons. The Hamar Clinics are envisioned to deliver free, accessible, continued and quality primary and preventive health-care facilities to all residents, including free consultation/counselling, examination/testing, medicines and health education, to reduce the overall out-of-pocket expenditure on health.

It is crucial that the service delivery and timing of the Hamar Clinic is centred around the working urban population. Thus, it is imperative that evening outpatient services are embedded in the culture of these centres.

The following services are to be delivered:

- Medical Consultation (MBBS) including compulsory evening OPDs. To develop the concept of a family doctor/physician.
- Medical Pharmacy
- Antenatal Care & Immunization
- NCDs: Routine Check-ups, timely screening, treatment & continued care.
- Sample Collection for Pathology Tests (through Hamar Labs)

- Community Outreach, Health Education & Awareness
- Addressal of the social determinants of health in the locality
- Referral support to higher centres and to ensure that there is no out-of-pocket expenditure on transportation
- Eye Clinic (Desirable)

Around 400 Hamar Clinics are planned across Chhattisgarh in the first phase of implementation.

B. Hamar Aspataal

The second tier of the urban health system would be the Hamar Aspataals, positioned over the Hamar Clinics, catering to a population of 50,000-75,000 persons, also with evening out-patient services embedded in their culture.[9] The Hamar Aspataal should be the first referral unit for the Hamar Clinics, and should provide patients with:

- Specialist Consultation
- Diagnostics Services (Pathology & Radiology)
  - o   In-House Pathology & Spoke to the Mother Hamar Lab
  - o   X-Ray, USG
  - o   Cancer Screening (Desirable)
- Inpatient Services
- Delivery (Labour) Services with Model Labour Rooms
- Basic Surgical Procedures (Fixed Day with Visiting Surgeons)
- Dental (Oral Health) Services
- Eye Clinic
- Mental Health Counselling
- Pain & Palliative Clinic
- Day Care Chemotherapy
- Day Care Peritoneal Dialysis
- Physiotherapy (Physical Medicine & Rehabilitation)
- Ayush Services & Wellness Activities

Four model Hamar Aspataals were set up in Raipur in 2020. Tata Trust has supported the initiative with funds for a model immunization room, IT system and internal branding. A total of 52 Hamar Aspataals are sanctioned across Chhattisgarh in the first phase of implementation.

Hamar Lab

Another important health-systems area where the state has made a start but is in early stages is of essential diagnostics in public facilities. It aims to do so through developing in-house capacity. Model laboratories have been operationalized in some of the district hospitals under the 'Hamar Lab' (Our Lab) initiative. A roadmap has been created to develop these services at various levels, including CHCs and urban PHCs.

To ensure uniform pathology services across the state, Hamar Labs are envisioned as the hubs to provide services through the hub and spoke model,[10] as recommended in the National Free Diagnostics Guidelines 2017. Hamar labs are envisioned at the following levels:

- Sample Collection & Point of Care Diagnostics at Health & Wellness Centres (PHC & SHC)
- FRU/Block Level Labs/ Integrated Public Health Labs
- Urban Public Health Labs
- District Hospital Mother Labs
- Medical College Specialized Labs

Model District and Block Level Labs have been set up and Medical College Labs are under construction.

Haat Bazaar Clinics

The Mukhyamantri Haat Bazaar Clinic Yojna was launched on 2 October 2019 with an aim to increase access to comprehensive primary health-care services in rural areas. Haat bazaars or weekly community markets have traditionally been locations where people from remotest of villages, especially in tribal areas, come to purchase items of sustenance. Thus, it was envisioned to bring primary health services to these locations to cater to populations relatively left underserved.

A team of medical professionals, led by an MBBS doctor, visited the earmarked 35,879 Haat Bazaars across the state on prescribed days of the month to establish a mobile clinic at these Haat Bazaars. These Haat Bazaar clinics provide basic medical consultations including eye, ear and dental checks and provide sixty-five types of medicines and fourteen types of kit-based tests for diagnostics. Those requiring further investigations or specialist care are referred to Community Health Centres or District Hospitals for further treatment.

Till August 2022, a total of 23,65,650 persons were provided medical consultation across 35,879 Haat Bazaars in Chhattisgarh.

Malaria Mukt Chhattisgarh Abhiyan

To address the health hazards of malaria, it was decided to conduct community-based active screening and complete treatment of all those found positive. Screenings took place in seven districts of Bastar division initially and all malaria-endemic districts of the state later, to reduce malaria parasite load. In these areas, malaria is also the main cause behind anaemia and malnutrition. Therefore, one of the related objectives of the Abhiyan is to reduce anaemia, maternal and child deaths as well as malnutrition. Reduction of malaria prevalence in such areas will also lead to improvement in socio-economic conditions of the tribal community, as it will lead to less expenditure on morbidity and also prevent wage loss.

Since January 2020, by end-2021, five rounds of this Abhiyan were carried out in Bastar division and two rounds in other districts. During the Abhiyan, not only are door-to-door visits made to all households in the endemic areas, but screening is also carried out in schools, ashrams, portable cabins and paramilitary camps so that nobody is left out. Those who are found positive, even if asymptomatic, are given treatment right away and 100 per cent compliance with the treatment is monitored by Mitanins[11] (initial version of the ASHA workers), who collect empty blister packs from those found positive during screening. Treatment cards are also provided to all such people who are found positive for follow-up later.

Post the first round of Abhiyan, UNICEF carried out independent third-party verification.[12] The results were quite encouraging: it found 91.30 per cent population coverage and completion of treatment in 95 per cent cases.

The initiative has resulted in a number of benefits:

- The test positivity rate for malaria during the Abhiyan has decreased from 4.60 per cent to 0.79 per cent.
- Annual malarial parasite incidence declined from 2.63 in 2018 to 0.92 in 2021.
- There has been a 62 per cent decline in malaria cases in 2021 in comparison to 2018.

Innovations in Health Human Resources

Human Resources (HR) for health is one of the major challenges in Chhattisgarh, with retention of doctors and health-care workers a big issue. Despite several efforts, by 2018 the availability of specialists was only 13 per cent and medical officers only 56 per cent against sanctioned posts. Due to concerted initiatives, this has now increased to 26 per cent for specialists and 95 per cent for medical officers, reducing the shortage against sanctioned posts from over 40 per cent to 5 per cent in the case of the latter. In order to tackle the shortfall of specialists, a one-time relaxation in the recruitment policy has been done to allow for direct recruitment of specialists in up to 50 per cent of the sanctioned posts.

In 2020, Chhattisgarh became the first state in the country to carry out the Health Labour Market Analysis (HLMA). The state roped in the World Health Organization (WHO) to carry out this important analysis, which examined both the supply-side as well as demand-side issues regarding human resources for health. The report entailed recommendations and solutions to two key policy questions: the sufficiency and efficiency of production of health workers to meet current demand and factors in relation to successful roll-out of health and wellness centres in the state.[13] The analysis provided the government a clear picture of what needed to be done to strengthen availability and quality of HR in the public system.

The HLMA cited issues like that of unmet special care needs due to unavailability of specialists on the demand side. On the side of supply was the lack of coherent administration procedures for Assistant Medical Officers (AMOs), inefficiencies in the recruitment process, concern for quality standards in education and training and excess production of nurses leading to poor remuneration and unemployment. It recommended alternative/diploma training courses, task-shifting, improving recruitment process of medical officers and specialist doctors, making the process of recruitment transparent for nurses, improving supportive services and other benefits to improve retention in remote areas, improving administration and capacity of AMOs, improving accreditation and quality-control mechanisms for all educational institutions and reducing the salary gap between contractual and regular nurses.

The state has started implementing these recommendations in terms of improving the quality of nursing education, initiating a postgraduate diploma course in Family Medicine, increasing attractiveness of government service through non-financial incentives such as ensuring housing, hostels, children's education, opportunities for spouses and PG education. Another important step has been the changes in doctors' recruitment rules and systems.[14] The state has reached very close to filling all the vacancies in positions of medical officers, staff nurses, laboratory technicians, ANMs and multi-purpose workers. Improving recruitment of specialist doctors remains a challenge and the state has a roadmap to overcome it.

The state had previously implemented the Chhattisgarh Rural Medical Corps (CRMC), another significant innovation for improving retention as well as attracting human resources for tribal and difficult areas. Through the CMRC, the state provides a block headquarters-based health department colony, transport facilities to peripheries, insurance schemes and study support for kin, in addition to the regular salary. With such incentives in place, more personnel are attracted to operationalize the PHCs in these medically un-served areas 24/7.[15]

The Rural Medical Assistant (RMA) cadre consisting of diploma clinicians has been another useful innovation in health HR. This cadre is trained specifically to manage primary care. The course for the training of RMAs is a three-year diploma in Modern and Holistic Medicine, consisting of the same allopathic texts that are studied in an MBBS degree programme. The trainees also undertake a year-long internship that includes a month of training at a sub-centre, three months at a Primary Health Centre (PHC), four months at a Community Health Centre (CHC) and four months of rotational posting at a District Hospital. The RMA posts are sanctioned at PHCs in remote or tribal districts, with female RMAs posted in remote Community Health Centres that lack female doctors. Unlike medical officers, RMAs are prohibited from independent practice.[16]

RMAs help in implementing national and state-level health programmes, providing preventive health care, primary health-care services and referrals, basic maternal and child health care, conducting deliveries, managing pregnancy complications and childbirth and suturing first-degree perineal tears. They can also perform services like simple operative procedures, repairing wounds by stitching, draining abscesses, dressing burns, applying splints in fracture cases and applying tourniquets in case of severe bleeding. They are, however, not permitted to be involved in medico-legal cases and perform post-mortems.

The skills of RMAs have been evaluated and found on par with medical officers when applied for services needed at PHC level. Studies that explored the much-debated ability of AYUSH doctors and RMAs to provide health care in the context of non-availability of medical officers trained in Western medicine at PHCs arrived at the conclusion that, even without formal training in clinical care, there is no significant difference in the performances of RMAs against physicians when it comes to history-taking, physical examination and correct prescription.[17] The scholar Var Ghese further states that even with the so-called sub-standard care for the rural population, the rural cadre has brought about justice through equity in the health-care system.[18]

It is true that political vision and ideologies of different ruling parties at different points of time influenced the government agenda on RMA option in health policy.[19] Nonetheless, the introduction of RMAs was a game changer in the state's health-care services where both the need for care and opportunity for employment are being met. However, with its diploma-holders demanding recognition as a doctor and the Medical Council of India raising legal issues, the government later had to withdraw this course altogether. The earlier trained RMAs continue in service.

Community-Based Initiatives Pioneered by Chhattisgarh

Realizing the importance of community engagement, the Chhattisgarh government has initiated several community-based programmes. Mitanin is one such programme, wherein a health volunteer who belongs to the same village and understands the local problems engages with the community in the local dialect.

Fulwaris, Mahila Arogya Samitis and Swastha Panchayat Yojana are other initiatives born as urgent responses to the public health crisis.

The Mitanins

Mitanins have three important roles—providing health education to communities along with care for simple ailments, linking them to formal health-care services and, as health activists, demanding better services.[20]

The Mitanin programme has contributed immensely to the positive outcome in infant and child mortality rate, maternity care, child immunization and vitamin A supplementation, child feeding practices and overall nutritional improvement. The initial success of the programme was in reproductive and child health indicators including aspects like immunization coverage, antenatal care coverage, institutional deliveries, oral rehydration for diarrhoea, early initiation of breastfeeding and child nutrition, with significant improvements in terms of women's nutrition and anaemia. The next set of issues that Mitanins have impacted is disease control, most notably malaria, newborn infections and Acute Respiratory Illnesses (ARIs) in children. Mitanins play a central role in identification and referrals for TB and leprosy as well. Some of the new areas on which Mitanins are working now include:

- Dengue prevention in urban slums
- Testing of drinking water to check for contamination
- Counselling of parents for psycho-social development of young children
- Promotion of community-managed child care centres (called 'Fulwaris') for holistic development of children encompassing elements of health, nutrition and care
- Follow-up of NCDs, especially hypertension cases and sickle-cell patients
- Anti-tobacco campaigns, especially among adolescents

The key advantages Mitanins offer are of their proximity to the community and the credibility they enjoy. Their skills have improved with repeated trainings, and they are the prime movers in promoting collective community action on prevention and promotion aspects of health. An effective training and support system, which has contributed to an ongoing increase in their health skills, has enhanced the Mitanins credibility in the community, which in turn helps their work as activists and organizers of the community. Indeed, social recognition and a desire to learn new things remain the key motivators for the Mitanins and Chhattisgarh has adopted these strategies well. The ASHA programme under the National Rural Health Mission was adopted based on the Mitanin model.

To increase the availability of trained nurses, especially in remote areas, and provide a career-advancement path to the Mitanins, the Chhattisgarh government initiated a career development programme for Mitanins under the National Rural Health Mission (NRHM). Those having a Class-12 qualification in the science stream were sponsored by NRHM for a BSc in Nursing. In 2010, Mitanins were sponsored for Auxiliary Nurse Midwifery (ANM) courses in private ANM schools. These Mitanins then filled the vacant ANM posts in backward districts. By 2011, the government had this initiative institutionalized, reserving 40 per cent of seats in government ANM training schools.

Mitanin Online Incentive Payment System

The NHM guidelines have provisions for performance-based incentives for Mitanins. However, ensuring timely payment of their incentives under various national programmes has always been a challenge. To address the issue, a web-based solution has been drafted, which will have three major functions:

• Recording the performance of Mitanins.

- Seamless incentive disbursement system without any additional resource burden on the state while providing a monitoring mechanism for the same to state-level authorities.
- Administrative management of data for planning and budgeting.

The Mitanin Incentive Online Payment System (MIPS) facilitates timely and seamless online incentive payment to Mitanins directly into their bank accounts. It also captures Mitanin-wise details of services given to the community and generates reports to monitor progress. The system has proven to be one of the most user-friendly tools for the ground-level workforce as well. Till January 2022, Rs 569 crore has been paid towards Mitanin incentives.

The Fulwaris

The Fulwari programme was incorporated in the Chhattisgarh health-care system as a community-managed nutrition-cum-day-care. Groups of caregivers manage Fulwari centres with funds from the government that they receive through local elected bodies. Mitanins carry out the tasks of community mobilization and capacity building. The meals provided include adequate calorie-dense vegetables and eggs procured locally. These day-care centres compensate for the shortage of caregiver time in families and recurrent infections resulting from inadequate diet.[21]

Mahila Arogya Samitis and Swastha Panchayat Yojana

Yet another initiative for helping the Mitanins in the planning for provision of health-care services is that of Mahila Arogya Samiti (MAS). MAS assists Mitanins in spreading awareness about different health-related government schemes to the poorest and most backward regions in the state.[22] These are members from the same community who are aware about the local health issues and can suggest the best possible solutions.

Swastha Panchayat Yojana, initiated by the Department of Health and Family Welfare, Chhattisgarh, with the assistance of the State Health Resource Centre (SHRC), aims for a panchayat agenda to accommodate health and action on health-related issues. A survey based on a set of ten panchayat-level indicators, namely, health status, access to health-care services, health-related community behaviour, nutrition, education, water and sanitation and gender is carried out. The objectives of the Swasthya Panchayat Yojana include enabling the communities and panchayat members to know and assess the status of health at the *gram* level, ranking panchayats in order of their composite performance and identifying specific weak areas in terms of defined indicators, facilitating stakeholder dialogue, and encouraging panchayats to draw up and implement a participatory plan to improving health status of the gram.[23]

The Suposhan Abhiyaan

The NFHS data from rounds three and four shows improving figures in nutrition indicators. Children under five years who are underweight, for instance, have reduced from 47.1 per cent (2005–06) to 37.7 per cent (2015–16). Yet, this leaves much to achieve. The state has been proactive in meeting this challenge. In addition to the Fulwaris, in 2019, the Chhattisgarh government launched the Mukhyamantri Suposhan Abhiyaan (Chief Minister Nutrition Scheme), with the help of panchayats and self-help groups.[16] It provides for hot nutritious cooked food to malnourished children and anaemic women after a pilot in three districts demonstrated benefits of this initiative.[24]

Public-Sector Infrastructure and Institutional Engineering

In addition to the people-oriented health facilities and models that the state has come up with, it has attempted to strengthen the institutional capacity, with 'governance decisions' executed in a way that strengthens the public sector infrastructure. Drug procurement systems, the State Health Resource Centre and AYUSH services have been developed to ensure proper health care and community-centric treatment. Medical education and training too have been widened to accommodate the shortfalls of human resource in health-care facilities.

Drug Procurement and Distribution System: Setting Up of the CGMSCL

Chhattisgarh became the first state in India to publish its own essential drug list (EDL) enlisting the standard treatment guidelines and state drug formulary. The state was looking to solve the pertinent drug access problem by ensuring availability of free generic medicines in government hospitals.

Therefore, the Chhattisgarh Medical Services Corporation Limited (CGMSCL) was set up to conduct the procurement and distribution of drugs and other medical supplies. It depends upon indents received from Directorates of Health Services (DHS) and Medical Education (DME), based on the demands of their respective hospitals and medical colleges, to purchase drugs and initiate rate contracts (purchase contracts valid for two years). As the indenting mechanism of both DHS and DME is not reflective of the actual drug consumption, the inaccurate indents resulted in an inefficient purchase strategy by CGMSCL and absence of rate contracts for essential medicines.

Thus, it was decided that for items on the Essential Drug List, irrespective of an indent from DHS or DME, there should always exist a valid rate contract with CGMSC. It was also decided that every facility, based on the facility type, should at all times have a minimum stock of items listed in the EDL. In case the stock fell below the threshold, CGMSC should push stock from their warehouse to ensure that the minimum stock levels were maintained in each facility. In case of shortage of stock at warehouse, inter-facility transfer of stock from a surplus facility to a deficit facility may be considered.

Epitomizing Primary Health Care through Health and Wellness Centres

Chhattisgarh was a pioneer in initiating Health and Wellness Centres. Jan Swasthya Sahayog (JSS), an NGO in Chhattisgarh, developed a model of organizing primary-care services in Bilaspur district. It was followed by experiments in the government sector in Korba district in 2016–17. HWCs went on to become part of national policies, with the first formal HWC inaugurated in Chhattisgarh. To be able to start the HWCs quickly, Chhattisgarh deployed its Rural Medical Assistants (RMAs) to run clinics in HWCs. Currently, Chhattisgarh has nearly 2000 HWCs. These centres provide care for a wide range of primary health care needs including NCDs. Nurses are being trained as Community Health Officers and the state is on its way to converting all its 5200 Sub-Health Centres into HWCs over the coming two to three years, expanding the range of services to include tele-medicine, wellness activities, community outreach, etc.

Civil Society Partnerships and Institutional Innovation

Chhattisgarh has been fortunate to have some of the most innovative civil society organizations in the health sector. The state has been engaging with these institutions in the non-profit sector by empanelling NGO hospitals as providers of health care under its Trust Model. But beyond utilizing their services in implementing programmes, the state has really benefited by using the innovative experiences of civil society and adopting models developed by it. The Fulwaris and HWCs, which have been built on the Jan Swasthya Sahayog models, mentioned above, are key examples.

Civil society has also been engaged in capacity building of health HR in the public sector. The State Health Resource Centre (SHRC) is an important institutional innovation. This is an autonomous society created in collaboration with civil society in 2002 to serve two main functions: a) to manage the Mitanin and related community-based initiatives, and b) to provide analysis, advice and support for strengthening health systems in Chhattisgarh. The SHRC backed the Mitanin programme by assisting in finalization of the model, designing a social mobilization campaign for community involvement in the public health system and a media and communications strategy for the same. It assisted in developing and coordinating organizational details and implementation schedules for the programme, its training modules and pedagogy, and monitoring and evaluation systems.[25]

The SHRC is a unique organization in terms of its autonomous structure. The autonomy allowed in its operations has been the key to a successful Mitanin programme, as well in its providing credible feedback on other programmes. A team at the SHRC, comprising six programme coordinators and sixteen field coordinators, headed by a director, has been developed for successful implementation of its objectives. This team constantly interacts with the district and block levels. A nodal officer is appointed for this purpose who coordinates the district Mitanin coordination committee and the full-time district training teams which conduct the programme on a day-to-day basis.[18] A block medical officer or an NGO conducts the programme at the block level. At the village level, the gram panchayat endorses the Mitanin selection.

In 2006, the National Health Systems Resource Centre (NHSRC) was created at the national level under the National Rural Health Mission (NRHM), for which SHRC, Chhattisgarh, was a key reference. Today, at least thirteen states have an

operational State Health Resource Centre/State Health Systems
Resource Centre (SHRC/SHSRC).

MEDICAL PLURALISM

Chhattisgarh has also been the forerunner in taking programme
initiatives in AYUSH and the tribal/local health traditions. Special
effort has been made to provide people choice in health-care
knowledge systems and ensure the benefits of medical pluralism
reach all. A separate Directorate of AYUSH was created at the state
level for provisioning of AYUSH care in rural and urban areas.
Chhattisgarh was, in fact, found to be the highest AYUSH-utilizing
state in the country.[26] Various villages have been designated as
Ayurveda grams, under which Ayurveda dispensaries have been
established. Ayurveda-based lifestyles are promoted through yoga,
behavioural change and other wellness activities offered at Health
and Wellness Centres.[27] AYUSH doctors have been appointed in
the stand-alone AYUSH dispensaries and in the co-located general
health services.

Traditional healers have been identified to promote the local
traditional healing system. *Sirha-Guniya sammelans* have been
organized to identify these local traditional healers and bring
them into the mainstream of health-care delivery systems. The
Traditional Healer Association, Chhattisgarh, focuses on the
usage of traditional medicinal plants to meet modern needs and
encourages the villagers to do the same.[28] In the process, more than
one million medicinal plants and trees have been planted in 100
villages, 'restoring rare and threatened flora and fauna, improving
local health and livelihoods in the process'. The association works
closely with more than 1200 traditional healers to provide health-
care services to the rural population of the state. Recognizing
the value of these healing practices and healers, in 2020, the state
government renamed the Chhattisgarh State Medicinal Plant Board
as the 'Chhattisgarh Adivasi Sthaniya Swasthya Parampara Evam

Aushadhi Padap Board' (Chhattisgarh Tribal Local Health Tradition and Medicinal Plant Board) for promotion of medicinal plants and their utilization as per traditional local and tribal knowledge and practice and their continuing innovations.[29]

Dynamism and Adaptiveness

The state has been keen to adopt newer technologies and approaches to improve the dynamics of organization of health care. Aligning with various technology institutes like IITs, NITs, NIC, C-DAC, CHIPS and CREDA, the state has generated and adopted new methodological approaches for health systems strengthening. As evidenced by its partnerships with civil society and academic institutions of repute to introduce and moderate various policies, evaluate policy impacts as well as generate innovative solutions for access to and availability of health-care systems without financial hardship to the people, the state has made big strides, particularly in the last two years, in strengthening its public health system. The clarity of approach and ability to innovate has helped it in overcoming the barriers that often frustrate attempts to strengthen the health system. Most importantly, the innovations Chhattisgarh has devised are systemic and institutional in nature, with focus on community and public services, primary health care as well as hospital services. As opposed to being narrow and piecemeal, they are designed to be applied on scale and to have system-wide and long-term impact. This particular approach to innovations holds promise for Chhattisgarh and offers valuable lessons for all those outside the state interested in the practice of strengthening public systems. Many of its innovations have proved to be pioneering efforts which have been adapted for national-level application.

The overall health system of the state has improved in its efficiency as well as reach, making Chhattisgarh an example in terms of its innovative approaches towards the health rights of its population. The state has achieved UHC with its community-centric health systems solutions including that of the community health activists, the Mitanin model, the Haat Bazaar clinics, the Chhattisgarh Rural Medical Course (CRMC) and Rural Medical Corps,[23] which have helped access in medically underserved areas where doctors and other medical staff are not available to work. Simultaneously, the state has provided choices between available treatment options like that of traditional community health-care providers, AYUSH and allopathy. Expanding the social insurance scheme to all citizens and strengthening of public services has led to a shift in utilization from private to public services.

Innovations in governance structure and functioning have provided for the ongoing innovations in the service system, especially the collaboration with civil society. The State Health Resource Centre (SHRC) model provides a responsible and efficient structure that has effectively enacted a change in public health care through quality services and governance. The models of cadre development and service delivery developed by organizations such as Jan Swasthya Sahyog, the Leprosy Mission, Action Aid and Ramakrishna Mission Ashram have supported the community-and-public system approach of the Chhattisgarh government and its values of professionalism, integrity and ethics in health care.

The state understands that public health is not a responsibility of the health department alone; therefore, inter-sectoral and inter-departmental convergence has been taken on priority for planning and implementation of various public welfare schemes in the state. Nodal officers (inter-sectoral and inter-departmental convergence) have been appointed. Coordination with multiple stakeholders and community participation brings accountability and responsiveness in the system, for instance, through social audits conducted by the Village Health Sanitation and Nutrition committee members in rural areas and the Mahila Arogya Samitis in urban areas.

The government has time and time again stressed on public provisioning, discouraging the dependence on the private sector which works on the principle of profit maximization. The profit-seeking view invading the health-care system has been seen as an issue of serious concern by the Chhattisgarh government considering how private players have begun to influence public policies.[24] The Chhattisgarh Nursing Home Act has been implemented to maintain professionalism and ethics in the health system. To fix the accountability of service delivery within a reasonable time frame, some schemes of the health department have been included in the Lok Sewa Guarantee Adhiniyam. Workshops on rational use of drugs have been organized for health-care practitioners in collaboration with WHO and other agencies. The state has introduced exposure visits to field-level NGOs to orient medical students and interns, in which they have been trained on public health professionalism, integrity and ethics.

The COVID-19 pandemic did not deter the government from carrying out its activities for a 'malnutrition-free Chhattisgarh'. Under the Supplementary Nutrition Food Programme, ready-to-eat food items were distributed among under-six children, adolescent girls, pregnant and lactating women. Anganwadi centres and primary health-care services were reopened soon after the lockdown, with the view of continuity in prevention of malnutrition and mother and child health problems.

Though the health-care system in Chhattisgarh still faces several challenges, the hope is that the culture and vision the state has instilled within the health system structure, which is primarily based on a people-centred, inclusive and 'caring' governance, will continue fostering progress.

Notes

Introduction

1   India ranked 44 out of ninety-nine countries on the Global Health Care Index. This index is an estimation of the overall quality of the health care system, health care professionals, equipment, staff, doctors, cost, etc, https://www.numbeo.com/health-care/rankings_by_country.jsp However, it fared even worse in the Human Development Index ranking of 2019 that placed it at rank 131 out of 189 countries. https://hdr.undp.org/sites/default/files/hdr2020.pdf

Similarly, India's ranking of 101 out of 116 countries for the Global Hunger Index 2021, shows the low status relative to the high income and several low- and middle-income countries. The GHI is composed of indicators of inadequate food supply, child stunting and wasting, and child mortality, giving a summary index of health status of the population as well. https://www.globalhungerindex. org/about.html

We also have the triple burden of communicable, non-communicable diseases and injuries, at an extremely high level.

The worst is the ranking of the World Happiness Report 2021, where India stands at 139 out of 149 for the period 2018–20: https:// happiness-report.s3.amazonaws.com/2021/WHR+21.pdf, p. 23.

2   Margaret, E. Kruk, Anna, D. Gage, Naima, T. Joseph, Danaei, Goodarz, García-Saisó, Sebastián, Salomon, Joshua A., 'Mortality due to low-quality health systems in the universal health coverage era:

245

A systematic analysis of amenable deaths in 137 countries', *Lancet*, Vol. 392, Issue 10160, pp. 2203–2212, 17 November 2018 (https://doi. org/10.1016/S0140-6736(18)31668-4; last accessed on December 30, 2022 at 11:36 hours).

3   While corruption in health care is widely heard about in public discussion, medical journals and health analysts too have started to examine the problem of corruption in health care, as evident in the British Medical Journal campaign and publications. How they are addressing the issue can be seen for instance in: Anita Jain, Samiran Nundy, Kamran Abbasi, 'Corruption: Medicine's dirty open secret', BMJ, 2014, 348:g4184 DOI: 10.1136/bmj.g4184, https://www. bmj.com/content/bmj/348/bmj.g4184.full.pdf

The *British Medical Journal* took it up as a campaign, as stated in: Corruption in health care: https://www.bmj.com/campaign/ corruption-healthcare

Ritu Priya and Prachinkumar Ghodajkar, 'The Structural Basis of Corruption in Healthcare in India', and all the other papers in the book *Healers or Predators?: Healthcare Corruption in India*, Nundy, S., Desiraju, K., Nagral, S., eds, Oxford University Press, 2018, New Delhi, pp. 3–43.

4   'Closing the gap in a generation: Health equity through action on the social determinants of health', report of the Commission on Social Determinants of Health, WHO, 2008.

5   'Origin of SARS-CoV-2', WHO, 26 March 2020, https://apps. who.int/iris/bitstream/handle/10665/332197/WHO-2019-nCoV-FAQ-Virus_origin-2020.1-eng.pdf

6   Sara Platto, Jinfeng Zhou, Yanqing Wang, Huo Wang, Ernesto Carafoli, 'Biodiversity loss and COVID-19 pandemic: The role of bats in the origin and the spreading of the disease', Biochemical and Biophysical Research Communications, 538 (2021), 2e13.

7   World Health Organization-United Nations International Children's Emergency Fund, Declaration of Astana: Global Conference on Primary Health Care (Astana, Kazakhstan, 25–26 October 2018), Geneva, World Health Organization, 2018. 'Walking the Talk: Reimagining Primary Health Care after COVID-19' World Bank, Washington, DC, 2021.

India's Population Structure and Health Priorities of the Twenty-First Century

1   For discussions on explanations of fertility decline in India, see, Srinivasan, K., *Regulating Reproduction in India's Population: Efforts, Results, and Recommendations* (New Delhi: Sage, 1995), Kulkarni P.M., 2011, 'Towards an Explanation of India's Fertility Transition', *Demography India* 40(2):1–21.

2   All figures on population size and growth of India throughout the paper are from Table A-2 Decadal Variation in Population since 1901, Census of India, 2011, http://censusindia.gov.in/PCA/A2_Data_Table

3   Registrar General, India, *Sample Registration System Statistical Report, 2017* (New Delhi: Office of the Registrar General and Census Commissioner, India, Government of India, 2019).

4   United Nations, Department of Economic and Social Affairs, Population Division, 2022. *World Population Prospects 2022*, https://population.un.org/wpp

5   Vollset, Stein Emil, et al., 2020, 'Fertility, mortality, migration, and population scenarios for 195 countries and territories from 2017 to 2100: A forecasting analysis for the Global Burden of Disease Study', *Lancet*, published online on 14 July 2020, https://doi.org/10.1016/S0140-6736(20)30677-2).

6   The population percentages in 2011 by age and sex throughout the paper are computed from age-sex distribution of 2011 census, from Table C-13, https://censusindia.gov.in/2011census/DigitalLibrary/MFTableSeries.aspxTable C-13.html

7   The age distributions of projected population for India throughout the paper are computed from the tables of the Medium Variant of UN. World Population Prospects 2022, cited above.

8   United Nations, Department of Economic and Social Affairs, Population Division, *World Urbanization Prospects: The 2018 Revision, ST/ESA/SER.A/420* (New York: United Nations, 2019).

9   World Health Organization (WHO), 'Globalization, diets and noncommunicable diseases: Noncommunicable Disease Prevention and Health Promotion', cited 3 June 2014, http://whqlibdoc.who.int/publications/9241590416.pdf

10 Arellano, O.L., J.A.R. Marquez, V.I.D. Campos and J.B. Gil, 'Crisis living conditions and health in Mexico: New challenges for social policy', *Soc. Med*, 5, 2010, pp. 129–133.

11 Kahn, K., 'Dying to make a fresh start: Mortality and health transition in a new South Africa', 2006, Umeå University Medical Dissertations New Series No 1056, cited 18 August 2014, http://www.diva-portal.org/smash/get/diva2:145081/FULLTEXT01.pdf

12 Dilip, T.R., 'Understanding levels of morbidity and hospitalization in Kerala', *Bulletin of the World Health Organization*, 80, 2002, pp. 746–51.

13 Kennedy, G., Nantel, G., and Shetty, P., 'Assessment of the double burden of malnutrition in six case study countries', FAO Corporate Document Depository, www.fao.org.docrep/009/a0442e/90442e03.htm

14 Vellakkal, S., Subramanian, S.V., Millett, C., Basu, S., Stuckler, D. and Ebrahim, S., 'Socioeconomic inequalities in non-communicable diseases prevalence in India: Disparities between self-reported diagnoses and standardized measures', *PLoS One*, 2013, 8(7), e68219, 15 July 2013, doi:10.1371/journal.pone.0068219

15 Dhillon, P.K., P. Jeemon, N.K. Arora, et al., 'Status of epidemiology in the WHO South-East Asia region: Burden of disease, determinants of health and epidemiological research, workforce and training capacity' *Int. J. Epidemiol*, 2012, pp. 1–14.

16 'What share of people will live in urban areas in the future?', available at https://ourworldindata.org/urbanization#what-share-of-people-will-live-in-urban-areas-in-the-future

17 http://documents.worldbank.org/curated/en/878414564 98771492/Urban-health-advantages-and-penalties-in-India-overview-and-case-studies-discussion-paper

18 Atkinson, R., 'The flowing enclave and the misanthropy of networked affluence', chapter in *Blokland*, T., and Savage, M. (eds), *Networked Urbanism: Social Capital in the City*, Ashgate Publishing Ltd, 2008, pp. 41–58.

19 United Nations Department of Economic and Social Affairs/Population Division, World Urbanization Prospects: The 2011 Revision, retrieved from https://www.un.org/en/development/

desa/population/publications/pdf/urbanization/WUP2011_
Report.pdf

20   Ravallion. M., 'On the urbanization of poverty', *Journal of Development Economics*, 68, 2002, pp. 435–42.

21   Vearey J., 'Challenging urban health: Towards an improved local government response to migration, informal settlements, and HIV in Johannesburg, South Africa', Global Health Action, 4, 2011, 10.3402/gha.v4i0.5898. doi:10.3402/gha.v4i0.5898

22   Central Bureau of Health Intelligence, National Health Profile 2019, retrieved from https://cbhidghs.gov.in/showfile.php?lid=1147

23   CSDH, 'Closing the gap in a generation: Health equity through action on the social determinants of health' Final Report of the Commission on Social Determinants of Health, 2008, Geneva, World Health Organization.

24   McMichael, A.J., et al., 'Global environmental change and health: impacts, inequalities, and the health sector', *BMJ*, 336, 2008, pp. 191–94.

25   Editorial, 'Urban health post-2015', *Lancet*, 2015, retrieved from https://www.thelancet.com/action/showPdf?pii=S0140-6736%2815%2960418-4

Ensuring Health for All, in All Policies

1   Whitehead M., *The Concepts and Principles of Equity and Health* (Copenhagen: World Health Organization; 1990), p. 5.

2   Venkatapuram S., *Health Justice: An Argument from the Capabilities Approach* (Cambridge: Polity Press, 2011).

3   Kickbusch, I., Allen, L., Franz, C., 'The commercial determinants of health', *Lancet Glob Heal*, 2016, 4(12), pp. 895–6.

4   'Commission on Social Determinants of Health. Closing the gap in a generation: Health equity through action on the social determinants of health', Geneva, 2008, available at http://whqlibdoc.who.int/hq/2008/WHO_IER_CSDH_08.1_eng.pdf

5   Preston, S., 'The Changing Relation between Mortality and Level of Economic Development', *Popul Stud* (NY), 1975, 29(2), pp. 231–48.

6   Wilkinson, R.G., Pickett, K.E., 'Income inequality and population health: a review and explanation of the evidence', *Soc Sci Med*, 2006, 62(7), pp.1768–84, available at http://www.ncbi.nlm.nih.gov/pubmed/16226363

7   Kenny, P., 'Vaccine gap grows between rich and poor: WHO chief', Anadolu Agency, 22 March 2021, available at https://www.aa.com.tr/en/europe/vaccine-gap-grows-between-rich-and-poor-who-chief/2184613

8   Zimmerman, E., Woolf, S. HA, 'Understanding the Relationship Between Education and Health: A Review of the Evidence and an Examination of Community Perspectives', Rockville, 2015.

9   World Bank, World Development Report 2012 : Gender Equality and Development, 2012, available at https://openknowledge.worldbank.org/handle/10986/4391

10   Herman, D.R., Taylor Baer, M., Adams, E., Cunningham-Sabo, L., Duran, N., Johnson, D.B., Yakes E. Life, 'Course Perspective: Evidence for the Role of Nutrition', *Matern Child Health J*, 2014, 18, pp. 450–61.

11   Watts, B., 'The Dangers of Monoculture Farming', Challenge Advisory, 2018, cited 31 July 2021, available at https://www.challenge.org/knowledgeitems/the-dangers-of-monoculture-farming/

12   Elizabeth, L., Machado, P., Zinöcker, M., Baker, P., Lawrence M., 'Ultra-Processed Foods and Health Outcomes: A Narrative Review', Nutrients, 2020, 12(7), available at https://doi.org/10.3390/nu12071955

13   Shah, S., Magalhaes, L., Bariyo, N., 'Food Prices Soar, Compounding Woes of World's Poor', *Wall Street Journal*, 20 May 2021, https://www.wsj.com/articles/food-prices-soar-compounding-woes-of-worlds-poor-11621519202

14   Willett, W., Rockström, J., Loken, B., Springmann, M., Lang, T., Vermeulen, S., Garnett, T., Tilman, D., DeClerck, F., Wood, A., Jonell, M., Clark, M., Gordon, L.J., Fanzo, J., Hawkes, C., Zurayk, R., Rivera, J.A., De Vries, W., Majele Sibanda, L., Afshin, A., Chaudhary, A., Herrero, M., Agustina, R., M.C., 'Food in the Anthropocene: the EAT-Lancet Commission on healthy diets from sustainable food systems', *Lancet*, 2019, 393(10170), pp. 447–92.

15 Patterson, R., Webb, E., Millett, C., Laverty, A.A., 'Physical activity accrued as part of public transport use in England', *J Public Health* (Bangkok), June 2019, 1, 41(2), pp. 222–30, https://doi.org/10.1093/pubmed/fdy099

16 UN-Habitat, 'The Challenge of Slums: Global report on Human Settlements', London, Earthscan, 2003, http://www.loc.gov/catdir/toc/ecip045/2003013446.html

17 Lelieveld, J., Evans, J.S., Fnais, M., Giannadaki, D., Pozzer, A., 'The contribution of outdoor air pollution sources to premature mortality on a global scale', *Nature*, 2015, 525(7569), pp. 367–71, https://doi.org/10.1038/nature15371

18 Watts, N., Amann, M., Arnell, N., Ayeb-Karlsson, S., Belesova, K., Boykoff, M., et al, 'The 2019 report of the Lancet Countdown on health and climate change: ensuring that the health of a child born today is not defined by a changing climate', 2019, cited 1 August 2021, 394, https://doi.org/10.1016/

19 Heise, L., Greene, M.E., Opper, N., Stavropoulou, M., Harper, C., Nascimento, M., et al, 'Gender Equality, Norms, and Health 1 Gender inequality and restrictive gender norms: Framing the challenges to health', *Lancet*, 2019, 393, http://dx.doi.org/10.1016/

20 Langer, A., Meleis, A., Knaul, F.M., Atun, R., Aran, M., Arreola-Ornelas, H., et al, 'The Lancet Commissions Women and Health: the key for sustainable development', *Lancet*, 2015, 386, pp. 1165–210, http://dx.doi.org/10.1016/

21 Abel, G.J., Brottrager, M., Crespo Cuaresma, J., Muttarak, R., 'Climate, conflict and forced migration', *Glob Environ Chang*, 2019, 54, pp. 239–49, https://www.sciencedirect.com/science/article/pii/S0959378018301596

22 Whitmee, S., Haines, A., Beyrer, C., Boltz, F., Capon, A.G., Ferreira, B., et al., The Lancet Commissions The Rockefeller Foundation: Lancet Commission on planetary health Safeguarding human health in the Anthropocene epoch, report of The Rockefeller Foundation-Lancet Commission on planetary health, the Lancet Commissions, 2015, 386, pp.1973–2028, http://dx.doi.org/10.1016/http://www.thelancet.com/infographics/planetary-health

23   World Economic and Social Survey 2014/2015, UN, 2016, cited 2 August 2021, World Economic and Social Survey (WESS), https://www.un-ilibrary.org/content/books/9789210572705

24   WHO Report on the Global Tobacco Epidemic, 2011, the MPOWER Package, Geneva, 2011.

25   Global Panel on Agriculture and Food Systems for Nutrition, Food Systems and Diets: Facing the Challenges of the 21st Century, London, 2016, https://glopan.org/sites/default/files/ForesightReport.pdf

26   Willett, W., Rockström, J., Loken, B., Springmann, M., Lang, T., Vermeulen, S., Garnett, T., Tilman, D., DeClerck, F., Wood, A., Jonell, M., Clark, M., Gordon, L.J., Fanzo, J., Hawkes, C., Zurayk, R., Rivera, J.A., De Vries, W., Majele Sibanda, L., Afshin, A., Chaudhary, A., Herrero, M., Agustina, R., M.C., 'Food in the Anthropocene: The EAT-Lancet Commission on healthy diets from sustainable food systems', *Lancet*, 2019, 393 (10170), pp. 447–92.

27   Whitmee, S., Haines, A., Beyrer, C., Boltz, F., Capon, A.G., Ferreira, B., et al., report of The Rockefeller Foundation-Lancet Commission on planetary health, http://dx.doi.org/10.1016/http://www.thelancet.com/infographics/planetary-health

28   Rajan, D., Mathurapote, N., Putthasri, W., et al., 'Institutionalising Participatory Health Governance: Lessons from Nine Years of the National Health Assembly Model in Thailand', *BMJ Global Health*, 2019, 4:e001769.

A Scaffolding for Rebuilding Public Health Services in India

1   Winslow Charles-Edward Amory, Untilled field of public health, *Science*, 51(1306), 1920, pp. 23–33, https://zenodo.org/record/1448241#.X7yzdLPhXIU, accessed on 24 November 2020.

2   Institute of Medicine, 'The Future of Public Health', Washington, DC: The National Academies Press, 1988, https://doi.org/10.17226/1091, e-book accessed on 15.11.2020

3   WHO, Health System Financing: The Path to Universal Coverage, WHO, Geneva, 2010.

4   Qadeer Imrana, 'Political Economy of Knowledge: A Case of Primary Health Care in India', in Imrana Qadeer (series editors K.R.

Nayar and Rama Baru), *Public Health in India: Critical Reflections*, pp. 3–28, Daanish Books, 2011, New Delhi.

5   Mahalanobis, P.C., 'The Approach of Operations Research to Planning in India', *Sankhyā: The Indian Journal of Statistics* (1933–1960), Vol. 16, No. 1/2 (Dec.), p. 4, https://www.jstor.org/stable/25048270?seq=1, accessed on 2 November 2020.

6   Ibid., pp. 5–6.

7   Ibid.

8   Pathak Avijit, 'Searching for Glimpses of Nehru in a Parochial, Post-Nehruvian India', The Wire, 27 May 2017, https://thewire.in/history/searching-glimpses-nehru-post-nehruvian-india, accessed on 24 October 2020.

9   Kuriakose Francis, Deepa Kylasam Iyer, 'Nehru and the Welfare State: Examining the Idea of Welfare State in the Nehruvian Context', January, 2015, https://www.researchgate.net/publication/305618490_Nehru_and_the_Welfare_State_Examining_the_idea_of_Welfare_State_in_the_Nehruvian_context, accessed on 8 November 2020.

10   DeLong, J. Bradford, 'India Since Independence: Analytic Growth Narrative', 2012, https://www.researchgate.net/publication/246458096_India_Since_Independence_An_Analytic_Growth_Narrative, accessed on 24 October 2020.

11   Rao, A.V.V.S.K., 'Democracy and Development: Nehruvian Vision', *Mainstream*, 26 November 2017, www.mainstreamweekly.net/article7617.html, accessed on 10 September 2021.

12   GoI, Sixth Five Year Plan, Chapter I Development Performance, 1981, Planning Commission, New Delhi, https://niti.gov.in/planningcommission.gov.in/docs/plans/planrel/fiveyr/welcome.html, accessed on 22 October 2020.

13   Mahalanobis, P.C., 'The Approach of Operations Research to Planning in India', pp. 49, 77.

14   Sethuramalingam, V., Selwyn Stanley and Sathia, S., 'The Five Year Plans in India: The Overview of Public Policy', https://www.researchgate.net/publication/327238255_The_five_year_plans_in_India_Overview_of_Public_Health_Policies, accessed on 10 November 2020.

15 GoI, Report of the Committee on Health and Development (Bhore Committee), Vol. II, Delhi, Manager of Publications, 1946, p. 20.

16 George Mathew, 'The Fragmentation and Weakening of Institutions of Primary Healthcare, A Prescription for Their Revival', *Economic and Political Weekly*, Vol. 55, Issue No. 42, 17 October 2020, https://www.epw.in/journal/2020/42/special-articles/fragmentation-and-weakening-institutions-primary.html, accessed on 15 November 2020.

17 Chakravarthi, Indira, 'Universal Healthcare and Health Assurance through Healthcare Industry and Market Mechanisms: Evidence versus Ideology', in Imrana Qadeer, K.B. Saxena, P.M. Arathi (eds), *Universal Heathcare in India: From Care to Coverage*, Sage, New Delhi, pp. 74–97.

18 Leslie Charle, 'What caused India's massive community health workers scheme: A sociology of knowledge', *Social Science & Medicine*, Volume 21, Issue 8, 1985, pp. 923–30, accessed on 10 November 2020.

19 Sivaraman, B., 'Fair Wage Is a Question of Dignity for Anganwadis', Newspack, India Press Agency, 15 November 2020, https://ipanewspack.com/category/entertainment/, accessed on 15 November 2020.

20 Negandhi Himanshu, Kavya Sharma, Sanjay P. Zodpey, 'History and Evolution of Public Health Education in India', *Indian Journal of Public Health*, Vol. 56, Issue 1, 2012, pp. 12–16, https://www.ijph.in/article.asp?issn=0019-557X;year=2012;volume=56;issue=1;spage=12;epage=16;aulast=Negandhi, accessed on 13 November 2020.

21 Dongre Amol, R., Deshmukh, Pradeep, Swarup Garg, Bishan, 'An evaluation of ROME camp: Forgotten innovation in medical education', *Education for Health Change in Learning & Practice*, Vol. 23 (1), p. 363, April 2010, https://www.researchgate.net/publication/44853555_An_evaluation_of_ROME_camp_Forgotten_innovation_in_medical_education, accessed on 26 October 2020.

22 Srivastava, S., Fledderjohann, J., and Upadhyay, A.K., 'Explaining socioeconomic inequalities in immunisation coverage in India: New insights from the fourth National Family Health Survey (2015–16)',

BMC Pediatr 20, 295, 2020, https://bmcpediatr.biomedcentral.com/articles/10.1186/s12887-020-02196-5, accessed on 13 November 2020.

23 Jacob, Puliyel, 'Vaccine Policy of the Government of India: Driven and Controlled by Vested Interests?', in Imrana Qadeer, K.B. Saxena, P.M. Arathi (eds), *Universal Heathcare in India: From Care to Coverage*, pp. 287–310.

24 Mukhopadhyay, Indranil, 'National Health Policy 2015: Growth Fundamentalism Driving Universal Health Care Agenda?', *Universal Heathcare in India: From Care to Coverage*, pp. 98–116.

25 Ibid.

26 Ghosh, Sourindra Mohan and Qadeer, Imrana, 'An Inadequate and Misdirected Health Budget', The Wire, 8 February 2017, https://thewire.in/health/health-budget-2017-18, accessed on 12 November 2020.

27 Qadeer, Imrana and Ghosh, Sourindra Mohan, 'COVID-19: Beyond Biological Dynamics', *Social Change*, 24 July 2020, https://doi.org/10.1177/0049085720936076

28 Banerji, Debabar, 'A Vision for an Alternate Public Health Service for India', *Universal Heathcare in India: From Care to Coverage*, pp. 305–18, Sage.

29 Poulose, K.P., Natarajan, P.K., 'Re-orientation of medical education in India past, present and future', *Indian J Public Health*, Vol. 33, Issue 2, pp. 55–8.

30 Illich Ivan, *Medical Nemesis: Expropriation of Health*, Random House, 1975.

31 Nundy Samiran, Keshav Desiraju and Sanjay Nagral (eds), *Healers or Predators?: Healthcare Corruption in India*, OUP, New Delhi, 2018.

32 Banerji, Debabar, 'A Vision for an Alternate Public Health Service for India'.

33 Shukla, Abhay and Arathi, P.M., 'Challenges of Reclaiming Public Health System: Experiences of Community-Based Monitoring and Planning in Maharashtra', *Universal Heathcare in India: From Care to Coverage*, pp. 422–39.

34 Chowdhury, Jayeeta, 'Healer in the Hinterland', 2020, http://www.socialworkindia.in/profiles/yogesh-jain, accessed on 8 December 2020.

Innovation in India's Health Sciences: Three Pathbreaking Examples

1. Levine, Susan, *Medicine and the Politics of Knowledge: Beyond the Microscope*, 2013.

2   Nandy, Ashis, *The Intimate Enemy: Loss and Recovery of Self under Colonialism* (Delhi: Oxford University Press), 1983.

3   Shankar, Darshan, *The Unfinished Agenda of Modernization*, in Alvares Claude (ed.), *Multicultural Knowledge and the University* (Goa: Multiversity, 2014), pp. 120–27.

4   Valiathan, M.S., 'Ayurveda-biology: The First Decade', Proceedings of Indian National Science Academy, 82(1), 13–19, March 2016.

5   Priya, Ritu and Shweta, A.S., ResearchandMarkets.com, 2019; *Status and Role of AYUSH and Local Health Traditions under the National Rural Health Mission*, Government of India, National Health Systems Resource Centre, Ministry of Health and Family Welfare, 2010.

6   Report under publication: Shankar, Prasan, et al., 'An Ayurveda approach for the treatment of Pulmonary mycosis – A case report', IAIM Healthcare Center, Bangalore.

7   Sasi Kala, M., 'Siddha Medicine and Clinical Presentation of Dengue Fever at Tertiary Care Hospital of Chennai, Tamil Nadu, India', *International Journal of Advanced Ayurveda, Yoga, Unani, Siddha and Homeopathy*, Vol. 3, Issue 1, 2014.

8   Peterson, C., Lucas, J., John-Williams, L., et al., 'Identification of Altered Metabolomic Profiles Following a Panchakarma-based Ayurvedic Intervention in Healthy Subjects: The Self-Directed Biological Transformation Initiative (SBTI)', *Sci Rep* 6, 32609, 2016, https://doi.org/10.1038/srep32609

9   Ansari, M.A., Khan, Z., 'Use of local health traditions for prevention and cure of diseases by households in northern India', *MOJ Public Health*, 2018;7(6):393-398. DOI: 10.15406/mojph.2018.07.00273

10 Bodeker, Gerard, and Kariippanon, Kishan, 'Traditional Medicine and Indigenous Health in Indigenous Hands', Oxford Research Encyclopedia, Global Public Health, DOI:10.1093/acrefore/9780190632366.013.155

11   Kohlmeier, M., De Caterina, R., Ferguson, L.R., Görman, U., Allayee, H., Prasad, C., Kang, J.X., Nicoletti, C.F., Martinez, J.A., 'Guide and Position of the International Society of Nutrigenetics/ Nutrigenomics on Personalized Nutrition: Part 2 - Ethics, Challenges and Endeavors of Precision Nutrition', *J Nutrigenet Nutrigenomics* 2016;9:28-46. doi: 10.1159/000446347

12   Headey, D., Chiu, A., Kadiyala, S., 'Agriculture's role in the Indian enigma: help or hindrance to the crisis of undernutrition?', Food Secur, 1–16, 2012, http://dx.doi.org/10.1007/s12571-011-0161-0

13   Thow, A.M., Kadiyala, S., Khandelwal, S., Menon, P., Downs, S., Reddy, K.S., 'Toward food policy for the dual burden of malnutrition: an exploratory policy space analysis in India', Food Nutr, Bull, 37 (3), 261–274, 2016, http://dx.doi.org/10.1177/0379572116653863.

14   Govindaraj, P., Nizamuddin, S., Sharath, A., et al, 'Genome-wide analysis correlates Ayurveda Prakriti' *Sci Rep* 5, 15786, 2015, https:// doi.org/10.1038/srep15786

15   Banerjee, Subhadip, Debnath, Parikshit, Kumar Debnath, Pratip, 'Ayurnutrigenomics: Ayurveda-inspired personalized nutrition from inception to evidence', *Journal of Traditional and Complementary Medicine*, Vol. 5, Issue 4, October 2015, pp. 228–33.

16   Pingali, Prabhu, Mittra, Bhaskar, Rahman, Andaleeb, 'The bumpy road from food to nutrition security – Slow evolution of India's food policy', Global Food Security, Vol. 15, December 2017, pp. 77–84.

17   Zeevi, D., Korem, T., Zmora. N., Israeli, D., Rothschild, D., Weinberger, A., et al., 'Personalized nutrition by prediction of glycemic responses', Cell, 2015;163:1079–94.

     Westerman, Kenneth, Reaver, Ashley, Roy, Catherine, Ploch, Margaret, Sharoni, Erin, Nogal, Bartek, Sinclair, David A., Katz, David L., Blumberg, Jeffrey B., Blander, Gil, 'Longitudinal analysis of biomarker data from a personalized nutrition platform in healthy subjects', *Sci Rep*, 2018, 8: 14685.

     Guthrie, Nicole L., Carpenter, Jason, Edwards, Katherine L., Appelbaum, Kevin J., Dey, Sourav, Eisenberg, David M., Katz, David L., Berman, Mark A., 'Emergence of digital biomarkers to predict and modify treatment efficacy: machine learning study', *BMJ Open*, Vol. 9, Issue 7, 2019.

18 Droujinine, I.A., and Perrimon, N., 'Defining the interorgan communication network: systemic coordination of organismal cellular processes under homeostasis and localized stress', Frontiers in Cellular and Infection Microbiology, 3, 2013, doi:10.3389/fcimb.2013.00082

19 Kotas, M.E., and Medzhitov, R., 'Homeostasis, Inflammation, and Disease Susceptibility', Cell, 160(5), 816–827, 2015, doi:10.1016/j.cell.2015.02.010

20 Ramsay, R.R., Popovic-Nikolic, M.R., Nikolic, K., Uliassi, E., and Bolognesi, M.L., 'A perspective on multi-target drug discovery and design for complex diseases', Clinical and Translational Medicine, 7(1), 2018, doi:10.1186/s40169-017-0181-2

21 Tang, J., and Aittokallio, T., 'Network Pharmacology Strategies Toward Multi-Target Anticancer Therapies: From Computational Models to Experimental Design Principles', Current Pharmaceutical Design, 20(1), 23–36, 2014.

22 Hopkins, A.L., 'Network pharmacology: the next paradigm in drug discovery', Nature Chemical Biology, 4(11), 2008.

23 Valiathan, M.S., 'Ayurveda-Biology: The First Decade. Proceedings of Indian National Science Academy', 82(1), 13–19, March 2016.

Co-producing and Pluralizing Health Knowledge for Re-visioning Development

1 Life expectancy in the United States was over fifty years in the 1920s, over seventy-eight years in 2018. Official briefs in November 2018 show that for the second time in three years, the average life expectancy in the United States has actually gone down: https://www.cdc.gov/media/releases/2018/s1129-US-life-expectancy.html

'Throughout the 20th century, the UK saw significant increases in life expectancy . . . Yet while mortality rates continued to improve during the 2000s, since 2011 they have stalled, and for certain groups of the population, gone into reverse.' https://www.health.org.uk/publications/reports/mortality-and-life-expectancy-trends-in-the-uk?gclid=Cj0KCQjwuMuRBhCJARIsAHXdnqOPLjeMJmUQJuGO-s2-QpwFt-N7_Z76vCXtt8jjJv-7I6V_-RixmZUaAiF2EALw_wcB

2   Mittal, M., Bondre, V., Murhekar, M., Deval, H., Rose, W., Verghese, V.P., et al., 'Acute Encephalitis Syndrome in Gorakhpur', Uttar Pradesh, Clinical and Laboratory Findings, *Paediatric Infectious Disease Journal*, 2018, 37(11):1101–6.

3   Singh, A.K., Kharya, Pradip, Agarwal, Vikasendu, Singh, Soni, Naresh, P. Singh, Jain, Pankaj K., Kumar, Sandip, Bajpai, Prashant K., Dixit, Anand M., Singh, Ramit K., and Agarwal, Tanya, *J Family Med Prim Care*, 2020 July, 9(7): 3716–3721, 2020, doi: 10.4103/jfmpc.jfmpc_449_20

4   Express Webdesk, 'Gorakhpur hospital deaths: Yogi Adityanath, J.P. Nadda visit BRD as death toll rises to 72', *Indian Express*, 13 August 2017.

5   HSMI, HUDCO Chair and NIUA, 'Towns of India: Status of Demography, Economy, Social Structure, Housing, and Basic Infrastructure', New Delhi, NIUA, 2016.

6   Priya, R., Singh, R., Das, S., 'Health Implications of Diverse Visions of Urban Spaces: Bridging the Formal-Informal Divide' *Front, Public Health*, 7:239, 2019, doi: 10.3389/fpubh.2019.00239

7   The concept of peri-urban spaces has been widely accepted not only as a geographical location but as conceptualizing the interface between rural and urban features of economic activity, social composition and infrastructure. Governance, planning and service delivery tend to ignore such areas, as a growing literature shows:

    Randhawa, P., Marshall, F., 'Policy transformations and translations: lessons for sustainable water management in peri-urban Delhi, India', Environ, Plann C: Government Policy 32, 93–107, 2014, https://doi.org/10.1068/c10204

    Waldman, L., Bisht, R., Saharia, R., Kapoor, A., Rizvi, B., Hamid, Y., Arora, M., Chopra, I., Sawansi, K., Priya, R., Marshall, F., 'Peri-urbanism in globalizing India: A study of pollution, health and community awareness', *Int. J. Environ*, Res, Public Health 14, 980, 2017, https://doi.org/10.3390/ijerph14090980

    Dasgupta P., Dasgupta, R., 'Immunisation coverage in India: An urban conundrum', *Economic and Political Weekly* 50(21):19-22, 2015.

8   WHO and UN-Habitat, Global Report on Urban Health, 2016, Geneva, WHO.

9   Healthy Habitats have been easily understood as prerequisites for a healthy population. However, besides almost half our urban populations that lives under 'slum' conditions, increasingly poor quality of environment, social stress and violence have marred the Indian landscape. 'Healthy Cities' initiatives in various parts of the world have attempted to bring formal urban development and community efforts together. WHO, *Healthy Cities: Effective Approach to a Rapidly Changing World*, 2020.

Health care habitats have been consciously nurtured by community efforts in some pockets in India, spanning the rural-urban continuum. Visionary leadership and collective action made it possible. There are comprehensive approaches, as in Dayalbagh in Uttar Pradesh:

https://www.dei.ac.in/dei/edei/files/Dayalbagh%20as%20a%20 Healthcare%20Habitat-%20PRESS%20RELEASE.pdf

https://www.thestatesman.com/business/international-centre-for-agroecology-to-be-launched-in-new-jersey-usa-1503023935.html

Others limit initiatives to specific activities:

https://in.linkedin.com/company/deccan-development-society

http://www.ddsindia.com/www/default.asp

Singh Chandni, Mythili Madhavan, Jasmitha Arvind, Amir Bazaz, 2021. Climate change adaptation in Indian cities: A review of existing actions and spaces for triple wins. *Urban Climate*, Vol. 36, March 2021, 100783, https://doi.org/10.1016/j.uclim.2021.100783

10   Peri-urban conditions and efforts of citizens to improve them, including the poor, provide learnings, as much literature shows:

Marshall, F., Dolley, J., 'Transformative innovations in peri-urban Asia', Research Policy, 2018, https://doi.org/10.1016/j.respol.2018.10.007

Priya, R., Bisht, R., Randhawa, P., Arora, M., Dolley, J., McGranahan, G., Marshall, F., 'Local Environmentalism in Peri-Urban Spaces in India: Emergent Ecological Democracy?', STEPS Working Paper 96, STEPS Centre, Brighton, 2017, https://steps-centre. org/publication/local-environmentalism-peri-urban-spaces-india-emergent- ecological-democracy/

Marshall, F., Dolley, J., and Priya, R., 'Transdisciplinary research as transformative space making for sustainability: Enhancing pro-poor transformative agency in periurban contexts' *Ecology and Society*, 23(3):8, 2018, https://doi.org/10.5751/ES-10249-230308

11　Priya, R., Singh, R., Das, S., 'Health Implications of Diverse Visions of Urban Spaces: Bridging the Formal-Informal Divide', *Front, Public Health*, 7:239, 2019, doi: 10.3389/fpubh.2019.00239

12　National Council of Urban Indian Health, 'Evidence Based Practice and Practice Based Evidence: What are they? How do we know if we have one?', https://ncuih.org/ebp-pbe/

13　WHO, WHO's Strategy for Traditional Medicine 2014–2023, Geneva, World Health Organisation, 2013.

14　WHO, 'Everybody's business—Strengthening Health Systems to Improve Health Outcomes: WHO's Framework for Action', Geneva, World Health Organisation, 2007.

15　Ammerman, A., Smith, Tosha Woods, and Calancie, Larissa, 'Practice-Based Evidence in Public Health: Improving Reach, Relevance, and Results', *Annu. Rev. Public Health*, 35:47–63, 2014, doi: 10.1146/annurev-publhealth-032013-182458

16　Krieger, N., 'Theories for Social Epidemiology in the 21st Century: an eco social perspective', *Intern. J Epid.*, 30, pp. 668–77, 2001.

17　Sujatha, V., 'The Politics of Medicine in a Pandemic', *EPW*, Vol. LVI, No 30, pp.19–24, 2022.

18　World Health Organization, United Nations Children's Funds, 'Primary health care: Report of the International Conference on Primary Health Care', Alma-Ata, USSR, 1978, available via: https://apps.who.int/iris/handle/10665/39228, accessed on 14 October 2021.

19　The complexity of health systems requires dialogue across disciplinary, social identity, professional and layperson boundaries. See [6] and Priya, R., 'Critical Holism as Public Health Theory: Towards a Unifying Framework for Research, Policy and Planning', *Dialogue: Science, Scientists and Society*, Vol. 4, Special Issue on Public Health, 2021, DOI: https://doi.org/10.29195/DSSS.03.01.0033

20　Ghodajkar, P., Das, S., Sarkar, A., Gandhi, M.P., Gaitonde, R., Priya, R., 'Towards Reframing the Operational Design for HFA

2.0: Factoring in Politics of Knowledge in Health Systems', Medico Friend Circle Bulletin, No. 380, pp. 16–25, 2019.

21 Priya, R., 'AYUSH and Public Health: Democratic Pluralism and the Quality of Health Services', in Sujatha, V. and Abraham, L. (eds), *Medical Pluralism in Contemporary India,* Orient Blackswan, 2012, pp. 103–129.

Creating a System of Health-Care Providers for Universal Health Coverage

1 Muraleedharan, V.R., 'Professionalizing Medical Practice in Colonial South India', *EPW*, 1992.

2 Ibid.

3 Mudaliar, 'Health and Planning Committee', Government of India, 1961.

4 Ibid.

5 Kartat Singh Committee Report of 1972.

6 Shailaja Chandra, 'The Unqualified Medical Practitioners in India: The Legal, Medical and Social Dimensions of Their Practice', Shiv Nadar University, 2017.

7 'Chhattisgarh Experience with 3-Year Course for Rural Health Care Practitioners', a case study by Dr T. Sundararaman, Shomikho Raha, Dr Garima Gupta, Dr Kamlesh Jain, Dr K.R. Antony and Krishna Rao.

8 *Global Strategy on Human Resources for Health: Workforce 2030*, World Health Organization, 2016.

9 Ministry of Health, Government of India, August 2020.

10 DNB is Diplomate of National Board that by a gazette notification of the Government of India was made equivalent to the MD degree except for teaching purposes. The DNB is a degree conferred by the National Board of Examinations, an autonomous body set up in 1972, of the Ministry of Health and FW, GOI. The DNB candidates undergo three-year training in recognized hospitals, public and private, and have to pass a written examination.

11 The National Medical Commission Act of 2019.

The New Health-Care Paradigm: De-fragmenting Health-Care Systems

1 World Bank, Under-Five Mortality Rate, India, available at https://data.worldbank.org/indicator/SH.DYN.MORT?locations=IN
2 Wahl, B., Gupta, M., Erchick, D.J., Patenaude, B.N., Holroyd, T.A., Sauer, M., et al, 'Change in full immunization inequalities in Indian children 12-23 months: An analysis of household survey data', BMC Public Health, 2021, 21(1):841.
3 https://www.ncbi.nlm.nih.gov/pmc/articles/PMC8088616/
4 https://www.thehindu.com/sci-tech/science/23-million-children-in-india-unvaccinated-for-measles/article30231574.ece
   https://data.unicef.org/topic/child-health/immunization/
5 LBW: 18 per cent: https://bmcpediatr.biomedcentral.com/articles/10.1186/s12887-021-02988-3
   16 per cent: https://www.ijpediatrics.com/index.php/ijcp/article/view/4474/2856
6 World Bank, 'Traffic Crash Injuries and Disabilities: The Burden on Indian Society', Washington, DC, https://www.worldbank.org/en/country/india/publication/traffic-crash-injuries-and-disabilities-the-burden-on-indian-society
   https://www.thehindubusinessline.com/news/india-accounts-for-11-per-cent-of-global-death-in-road-accidents-world-bank/article33834556.ece
7 Tirupakuzhi Vijayaraghavan, B.K. NMS, Mathew, M., et al., 'Challenges in the delivery of critical care in India during the COVID-19 pandemic', Journal of Intensive Care Society, 2021.
8 Kaul, Rythma, 'More than 50% of heart attack cases reach hospital late, govt data shows', Hindustan Times, 2017, https://www.hindustantimes.com/india-news/more-than-50-of-heart-attack-cases-reach-hospital-late-govt-data-shows/story-penFdsewgGwpIwiQnRDoLJ.html
   https://timesofindia.indiatimes.com/city/mumbai/heart-attack-to-hospital-takes-6-hrs/articleshow/35579678.cms
9 Ministry of Health and Family Welfare, GoI, Non-communicable Diseases, 2019, https://www.nhp.gov.in/healthlyliving/ncd2019

10 Indian Council of Medical Research PHFoI, Institute for Health Metrics and evaluation, India, Health of the Nation's States: The India State-Level Disease Burden Initiative', New Delhi, India: ICMR, PHFI, IHME, 2017, https://www.healthdata.org/sites/default/files/files/policy_report/2017/India_Health_of_the_Nation%27s_States_Report_2017.pdf

11 John, O., Gummudi, B., Jha, A., Gopalakrishnan, N., Kalra, O.P., Kaur, P., et al., 'Chronic Kidney Disease of Unknown Etiology in India: What Do We Know and Where We Need to Go', Kidney Int Rep, 2021, 6(11):2743–51, https://www.ncbi.nlm.nih.gov/pmc/articles/PMC8589686/

12 'Mental health: India State-Level Disease Burden Initiative Mental Disorders Collaborators', *The Burden of Mental Disorders across the States of India: the Global Burden of Disease Study 1990-2017*, *Lancet Psychiatry*, 2020, 7(2):148-161. doi:10.1016/S2215-0366(19)30475-4

Building Equitable and Responsive Hospitals: Lessons from the Indian Experience

1   Government of India, Ministry of Statistics and Programme Implementation, National Statistical Office, Health in India, NSS 75th Round, July 2017 to June 2018, http://www.mospi.gov.in/sites/default/files/publication_reports/KI_Health_75th_Final.pdf

2   Apart from these hospitals, we also referred to the available literature on some other well-functioning secondary hospitals in the NGO sector—Makunda Christian Leprosy and General Hospital at Karimganj in Assam, and the Aravind Eye Hospital at Madurai, in Tamil Nadu.

3   Ministry of Health and Family Welfare, Government of India, National Health Policy 2017, https://www.nhp.gov.in/nhpfiles/national_health_policy_2017.pdf

Transforming Mental Health in India

1   Gururaj, G., Varghese, M., Benegal, V., et al, 'National Mental Health Survey of India, 2015-16: Summary', National Institute of Mental Health and Neuro Sciences, Bengaluru, 2016.

2   Patel, V., Ramasundarahettige, C., Vijayakumar, L., et al, 'Suicide mortality in India: A nationally representative survey', *Lancet*, 379(9834):2343–51, 2012.

3   Murthy, R.S., 'Mental health initiatives in India (1947–2010)', *Natl Med J India*, 24(2):98–107, 2011.

4   Shidhaye, R., Murhar, V., Gangale, S., et al., 'The effect of VISHRAM, a grass-roots community-based mental health programme, on the treatment gap for depression in rural communities in India: A population-based study', *Lancet Psychiatry*, 2017.

5   Patel, V., Weobong, B., Weiss, H.A., et al., 'The Healthy Activity Program (HAP), a lay counsellor-delivered brief psychological treatment for severe depression, in primary care in India: A randomized controlled trial', *Lancet*, 389(10065):176–85, 2017.

6   Patel, V., Saxena, S., Lund, C., et al., 'The Lancet Commission on global mental health and sustainable development', *Lancet*, 392(10157):1553–98, 2018.

7   Herrman, H., Patel, V., et al., 'Time for United Action on Depression: A Lancet-World Psychiatric Association Commission', 2022.

People over Profits: Reshaping India's Private Health Care

1   Farmer, Paul, *Pathologies of Power*, University of California Press, 2003.

2   'Measurement on the Healthcare Access and Quality Index for 195 Countries and Territories and Selected Subnational Locations: A Systematic Analysis from the Global Burden of Disease Study', *Lancet*, 23 May 2018, DOI: https://doi.org/10.1016/S0140-6736(18)30994-2

3   https://ficci.in/ficci-in-news-page.asp?nid=19199

4   Global Health Observatory Data, WHO, https://apps.who.int/gho/data/view.main.GHEDGGHEDGDPSHA2011WBv?lang=en

5   Hooda, S.K., 'Foreign Investment in Hospital Sector in India: Trends, Pattern and Issues', Working Paper No. 181, Institute for Studies in Industrial Development, New Delhi, April 2015.

6   Cleaton-Jones, I.P., 'Private Hospitals in Latin America: An Investor's Perspective', World Hospitals and Health Services, 2015, 51(2):7–9.

7   https://timesofindia.indiatimes.com/india/healthcare-for-poor-only-1-in-10-doctors-join-government-hospitals/articleshow/67239601.cms, accessed on 26 October 2020.

8   https://apps.who.int/iris/handle/10665/259642

9   https://www.hindustantimes.com/india-news/how-india-spends-on-health/story-CPyiZZ4jcI4imSKJq03jBM.html

10 Gadre, A., Shukla, A., *Dissenting Diagnosis*, Penguin India, 2016.

11 https://www.thehindu.com/news/national/spree-of-hysterectomies-to-make-a-fast-buck/article5007641.ece

12 Singh, Priyanka, et al., 'High prevalence of cesarean section births in private sector health facilities: Analysis of district level household survey-4 (DLHS-4) of India', *BMC Public Health*, Vol. 18, 1 613, 10 May 2018, doi:10.1186/s12889-018-5533-3

13 Sharma, R., 'Head of the Medical Council of India Removed for Corruption', *BMJ*, 15 December, 323(7326):1385. doi: 10.1136/bmj.323.7326.1385. PMID: 11744556; PMCID: PMC1121855.

14 Anand, S., Fan, V., 'The health workforce in India', Human Resources for Health Observer Series No. 16, Geneva, World Health Organization, 2016.

15 Hooda, S.K., 'Private sector in healthcare in healthcare delivery market in India: Structure, growth and implications', Institute for Studies in Industrial Development, New Delhi, 2015.

16 Marathe, S., Hunter, B.M., Chakravarthi, I., et al., 'The impacts of corporatisation of healthcare on medical practice and professionals in Maharashtra, India', *BMJ Global Health*, 2020, 5: e002026. doi:10.1136/ bmjgh-2019-002026

17 http://www.clinicalestablishments.gov.in/WriteReadData/5071.pdf

18 https://timesofindia.indiatimes.com/india/private-hospitals-making-over-1700-profit-on-drugs-consumables-and-diagnostics-study/articleshow/62997879.cms

19 Arrow, Kenneth, 'Uncertainty and Welfare Economics of Medical Care', *American Economic Review*, Vol. 53, Issue 5, December 1963.

20 https://www.newsclick.in/reforming-regulator-parliamentary-committee-report-medical-council-indi

21 https://scroll.in/article/956672/private-hospital-evicted-suspected-coronavirus-patient-alleges-chhattisgarh-government

22 Updhyay, A., 'Under Ayushman Bharat, huge disparities among states where Covid patients availed scheme', 16 June 2021, https://www.indiatoday.in/india/story/ayushman-bharat-huge-disparities-states-covid-patients-testing-treatment-1815303-2021-06-16

23 'Covid-19: Overcharging continues at Pune private hospitals during the second wave', *Times of India*, 5 June 2021, http://timesofindia.indiatimes.com/articleshow/83247505.cms?utm_source=contentofinterest&utm_medium=text&utm_campaign=cppst

24 Marpakwar, C., 'Mumbai: Private hospital Covid patients save Rs 15.5 crore, thanks to civic audits' *Times of India,* 18 March 2021, http://timesofindia.indiatimes.com/articleshow/81557285.cms?utm_source=contentofinterest&utm_medium=text&utm_campaign=cppst

25 More, D.M., 'Pimpri-Chinchwad: 76 private hospitals told to return Rs 6.44 crore overcharged to Covid patients', *Indian Express*, 16 June 2021, https://indianexpress.com/article/cities/pune/pcmc-committee-orders-76-private-hospitals-to-return-rs-6-44-crore-for-overcharging-covid-patients-7359639/lite/

26 https://nmji.in/first-national-conference-on-ethical-healthcare-nceh-2018-alliance-of-doctors-for-ethical-healthcare-adeh-all-india-institute-of-medical-sciences-new-delhi-21-22-april-2018/

27 https://www.hindustantimes.com/india-news/meet-the-man-who-fought-to-cap-coronary-stent-price-at-rs-30-000/story-8Nbn7MSAH1NBy17TZjJdUP.html

28 https://www.commonwealthfund.org/international-health-policy-center/countries/japan

29 Tangcharoensathien, V., Witthayapipopsakul, W., Panichkriangkrai, W., Patcharanarumol, W., Mills, A., 'Health systems development in Thailand: A solid platform for successful implementation of universal health coverage', *Lancet,* 24 March 2018, 391(10126): 1205–1223

30 Paek, Seung Chun, et al., 'Thailand's universal coverage scheme and its impact on health-seeking behavior', *SpringerPlus*, Vol. 5, 1 1952, 10 November 2016, doi:10.1186/s40064-016-3665-4

31 https://read.oecd-ilibrary.org/social-issues-migration-health/price-setting-and-price-regulation-in-health-care_ed3c16ff-en#page62

Redesigning and Revitalizing India's Public Health Governance: Addressing Abiding Antagonisms

1   Reports of corruption in the NRHM in Uttar Pradesh was extensively covered in the mainstream media and commented upon in public health literature on this period. See, for instance, Shubhalakshmi Shukla, 'India probes corruption in flagship health programme', *Lancet,* Vol. 379, 25 February 2012, p. 698, https://www.thelancet. com/journals/lancet/article/PIIS0140-6736(12)60293-1/fulltext

2   Krishnakumar, R., 'A better option in Kerala', *Frontline*, 12 April 2019, https://frontline.thehindu.com/cover-story/article26641511. ece

3   This data is available on the National Health Portal, https://chs.nhp. gov.in/AboutUs

4   See for example, Das Gupta, Monica, Desikachari, B.R., Somanathan, T.V., Padmanaban, P., 'How to Improve Public Health Systems: Lessons from Tamil Nadu', Policy Research working paper no. WPS 5073, World Bank, 2009, https://openknowledge.worldbank. org/handle/10986/4265; also, Parthasarathi, R., and Sinha, S.P., 'Towards a Better Health Care Delivery System: The Tamil Nadu model', *Indian Journal of Community Medicine*, October–December 2016, 41(4):302–304.

Innovations for Health Systems Strengthening in Chhattisgarh: A Public–Community Partnership

1   Insurance Regulator and Development Authority of India (IRDAI) chairman, T.S. Vijayan, gave an estimate of about 62 per cent of all health-care costs in India going out of pocket and showed how it was higher than even the developed countries. Special Correspondent, *The Hindu*, 18 December 2017, https://www.thehindu.com/ business/out-of-pocket-spend-makes-up-62-of-health-care-costs/ article21860682.ece

2   Government of India, *High Level Expert Group Report on Universal Health Coverage for India*, Planning Commission of India, New Delhi, 2011.

3   Ghose, D., T.S. Singh Deo interview: 'Ayushman scheme misleading . . . universal healthcare is a step ahead', *Indian Express*, 9 March 2019, https://indianexpress.com/elections/chhattisgarh-lok-sabha-elections-ts-singhdeo-interview-ayushman-scheme-misleading-universal-healthcare-is-a-step-ahead-5632859/, accessed on 18 October 2021.

4   Ibid.

5   Government of Chhattisgarh, Department of Health and Family Welfare and Medical Education, https://cghealth.nic.in/cghealth17/, accessed on 5 July 2021.

6   Nandi, S., 'Is the National Health Insurance Scheme in Chhattisgarh Doing More Damage Than Good?', The Wire, 3 November 2017, https://thewire.in/health/national-health-insurance-scheme-chhattisgarh-damage-good, accessed on 11 October 2021; Nundy, M., *The Rashtriya Swasthya Bima Yojana (RSBY) Experience in Chhattisgarh, What Does It Mean for Health for All?*, Sama: Resource Group for Women and Health, New Delhi, 2013, http://phrsindia.org/wp-content/uploads/2015/08/RSBY_Health-for-All_CG-experience.pdf; Shirisha, P., 'What Lessons should Pradhan Mantri Jan Arogya Yojana Learn from the Shortfalls of Rashtriya Swasthya Bima Yojana: The Case of Rashtriya Swasthya Bima Yojana in Chhattisgarh', *Indian Journal of Community Medicine*, 45, 2020, pp. 135–38, https://dx.doi.org/10.4103%2Fijcm.IJCM_95_19

7   https://dkbssy.cg.nic.in/

8   'Chhattisgarh government to start five new schemes on Gandhi Jayanti', *Business Standard*, https://www.business-standard.com/article/news-ani/chhattisgarh-government-to-start-five-new-schemes-on-gandhi-jayanti-119100100773_1.html, accessed on 22 October 2021.

9   Hamar Aspataal, NHM Innovations Summit, Chhattisgarh PPT, 19 January 2021, https://www.google.com/search?q=hamar+aspatal+bhatagaon&oq=Hamar+Aspatal&aqs=chrome.0.0i512j69i57j0i512j0i22i30i625l2j0i390l2.7355j0j15&sourceid=chrome&ie=UTF-8

10 'Chhattisgarh Government's "Hamar Lab": A Silent Change in Health Care', *Business Standard*, 4 July 2022, https://www.business-standard.

com/article/current-affairs/chhattisgarh-govt-s-hamar-lab-a-silent-change-in-health-care-122070401374_1.html; NHM Best Practices, Malaria Mukt Bastar Abhiyan, PPT, https://www.google.com/search?q=UNICEF+thrid+party+evaluation+of+malaria+chhattisgarh&sxsrf=AJOqlzUb-u2HFPtrXEQb3B8dj-GpVIIiug%3A1676165911820&ei=F0PoY7HPMcrhseMPwoGo4Ag&ved=0ahUKEwjxtojO7I79AhXKcGwGHcIACowQ4dUDCA8&uact=5&oq=UNICEF+thrid+party+evaluation+of+malaria+chhattisgarh&gs_lcp=Cgxnd3Mtd2l6LXNlcnAQAzIHCCEQoAEQCjIHCCEQoAEQCjoKCAAQRxDWBBBCwA0oECEEYAEoECEYYAFCNBVjpJ2CXRWgBcAF4AIABxwGIAegQkgEEMC4xM5gBAKABAcgBB8ABAQ&sclient=gws-wiz-serp, accessed on 22 July 2022.

11   State Health Resource Centre, 'Mitanin Programme in Chhattisgarh, India', http://www.cghealth.nic.in/cghealth17/Information/content/MediaPublication/MitaninProgrammedraft.pdf

12   NHM Best Practices, Malaria Mukt Bastar Abhiyan, PPT, https://www.google.com/search?q=UNICEF+thrid+party+evaluation+of+malaria+chhattisgarh&sxsrf=AJOqlzUb-u2HFPtrXEQb3B8dj-GpVIIiug%3A1676165911820&ei=F0PoY7HPMcrhseMPwoGo4Ag&ved=0ahUKEwjxtojO7I79AhXKcGwGHcIACowQ4dUDCA8&uact=5&oq=UNICEF+thrid+party+evaluation+of+malaria+chhattisgarh&gs_lcp=Cgxnd3Mtd2l6LXNlcnAQAzIHCCEQoAEQCjIHCCEQoAEQCjoKCAAQRxDWBBBCwA0oECEEYAEoECEYYAFCNBVjpJ2CXRWgBcAF4AIABxwGIAegQkgEEMC4xM5gBAKABAcgBB8ABAQ&sclient=gws-wiz-serp, accessed 22 July 2022.

13   World Health Organization, *Health Labour Market Analysis: Chhattisgarh*, India, World Health Organisation, https://cdn.who.int/media/docs/default-source/searo/india/publications/health-labour-market-analysis-9-july-2020.pdf?sfvrsn=52c4a4e4_2&download=true

14   https://cghealth.nic.in/ehealth/2017/DHS/2-MO-%20Gazted%20Bharti%20Niyam%202013.pdf

15   Chhattisgarh Rural Medical Course (CRMC), http://cghealth.nic.in/ehealth/CRMC.htm, accessed on 21 October 2021.

16 Jain, S., *Rural medical assistants in Chhattisgarh: Policy analysis and lessons for India*, master's thesis, Institute of Tropical Medicine Antwerp, Belgium, 2009–10, http://cgamoassociation.co.in/wp-content/uploads/2020/08/RURAL-MEDICAL-ASSISTANT.pdf

17 World Health Organization, *Health Labour Market Analysis: Chhattisgarh.*

18 Jain, S., *Rural medical assistants in Chhattisgarh: Policy analysis and lessons for India.*

19 Sarkar, A., 'People over Profit', *Deccan Herald*, 23 October 2018, https://www.deccanherald.com/opinion/main-article/people-over-profit-699470.html, accessed on 21 October 2021.

20 State Health Resource Centre, Mitanin Programme in Chhattisgarh, India.

21 Garg, S., 'Co-creating Nutrition Services through Community Managed Nutrition cum Daycare Centers – Fulwari Program from Chhattisgarh State of India' (Abstract), ACN2015 12th Asian Congress of Nutrition, Yokohama, 380, 2015, https://shsrc.org/wp-content/uploads/2020/04/FULWARI_ASIAN_NUTRITION_YOKOHAMA_JAPAN_MAY_2015.pdf; Srinivas, S., Fulwari Scheme in Chhattisgarh: A Case Study with Details for Replication. Centre for Innovations in Public Systems, Hyderabad, 2014, https://shsrc.org/wp-content/uploads/2020/04/A_CASE_STUDY_WITH_DETAILS_FOR_REPLICATION_CIPS_NOVEMBER_2014.pdf

22 State Health Resource Centre, Mahila Aarogya Samiti Formation MAS Guideline, https://shsrc.org/wp-content/uploads/2020/04/MAHILA_AAROGYA_SAMITI_FORMATION_MAS_GUIDELINE.pdf

23 State Health Resource Centre, Swastha Panchayat Guideline, https://shsrc.org/wp-content/uploads/2021/08/Swasth-Panchayat-Introduction-and-Methodology.pdf

24 https://shuposhitchhattisgarh.cgstate.gov.in/

25 https://shsrc.org/

26 Rudra, S., et al., 'Utilization of alternative systems of medicine as health care services in India: Evidence on AYUSH care from NSS', *PLoS One*, 12 (5), e0176916, 2017, https://www.ncbi.nlm.nih.gov/pmc/articles/PMC5417584/

27   Madhu, R., and Jain, N., 'Yoga Camoi in Ayurvedgrams of Chhattisgarh', *Journal of Ayurveda and Integrative Medicine,* 3(2), 2012, pp. 63–4, https://dx.doi.org/10.4103%2F0975-9476.96517

28   United Nations Development Programme, *Traditional Healer Association, Chhattisgarh, India,* Equator Initiative Case Study Series, New York, 2016, https://www.equatorinitiative.org/wp-content/uploads/2017/05/case_1471988205.pdf

29   'C'garh State Medicinal Plant Board Renamed', *National Herald,* 5 January 2021, https://www.dailypioneer.com/2021/state-editions/c---garh-state-medicinal-plant-board-renamed.html

About the Contributors

Abhay Shukla, a public health physician, is senior programme coordinator at SATHI-CEHAT. He is national co-convener of Jan Swasthya Abhiyan and a member of the Advisory Group on Community Action (AGCA). Dr Abhay has edited and co-authored several books, including *Review of Health Care in India*, *Report on Health Inequities in Maharashtra*, *Nutritional Crisis in Maharashtra* and *Dissenting Diagnosis* (published by Penguin). He has mentored the development of community-based monitoring and planning of health services in Maharashtra. He is engaged with campaigns for the regulation of private health-care sector, patients' rights, right to health care and initiatives for developing universal health care.

Anant Darshan Shankar is the vice chancellor of the Trans-Disciplinary University (TDU), Bangalore. Over the last twenty-five years TDU has inspired research and outreach in the field of Ayurveda–biology, a new transdisciplinary domain that combines systemic perspectives of Ayurveda with the molecular approaches of biology. His work has received several national and international awards, like the Norman Borlaug Award (1998), Columbia University's International Award (2003) for the revitalization of traditional systems of health care in India, and the Padma Shri, awarded by the Government of India in 2011.

C.N. Vishnuprasad, a postgraduate in biotechnology and PhD in cell biology, is currently working as associate professor at the Centre for Ayurveda Biology and Holistic Nutrition, TDU, Bangalore. He has more than fifteen years of research and teaching experience at universities in India and South Korea. Currently engaged in transdisciplinary research using the Ayurveda–biology framework for understanding the biology of glucose metabolism. He has several peer-reviewed research publications, conference papers and book chapters to his credit. He has been guiding PhD students at TDU and is also an advisory member for several PhD theses. He conceptualized and introduced an innovative transdisciplinary postgraduate programme, MSc life sciences (Ayurveda–biology), at TDU, and is one of the coordinators of this programme.

Gurmeet Singh is a scientist, inventor, innovator and entrepreneur with twenty-five-plus years of experience of working in academia and food industry research and development. He has a strong interest in 'food-first' solutions for health, wellness, equity and environment sustainability. Gurmeet has filed twenty-five patents, published twenty-five-plus articles and edited one book. He has a BTech in chemical engineering from Indian Institute of Technology Delhi and a PhD in chemical engineering from the Pennsylvania State University, USA. He spent four years in academia as a faculty of biochemical engineering at Penn State and IIT Delhi, and twenty years in Unilever, where he was the global R&D director for disruptive innovation. For the last five years, Gurmeet has been a professor at Trans-Disciplinary University in Bengaluru, where he heads the Centre for Ayurveda Biology and Holistic Nutrition. He has a keen interest in food futures and researches personalized nutrition, functional foods, plant proteins, food forests and tea processing.

Imrana Qadeer moved from paediatrics to public health and taught at the Centre of Social Medicine and Community Health, Jawaharlal

Nehru University, for thirty-five years. She then served as the J.P. Naik Senior Fellow at the Centre for Women's Development Studies and as distinguished professor at the Council for Social Development. Her areas of interest include organizational issues in health services in South Asia with a special focus on India, social epidemiology, and political economy of health, women's health and research methodology, with an emphasis on interdisciplinary research methodologies. She has also worked with the Ministry of Health and Family Welfare, the Planning Commission, Population Commission and the advisory bodies for the National Rural Health Mission. Among her publications is a selection of her research papers as a book titled *Public Health in India; Critical Reflections*, and the edited volumes *Public Health and the Poverty of Reforms: The South Asian Predicament* (2001), *CSD's Social Development Report – 2014: Challenges of Public Health* and *Universalising Healthcare in India: From Care to Coverage* (2019).

Kanchan Pawar is a physician and public health consultant working with SATHI, Pune. She is actively engaged in state and national campaigns for patients' rights and advocacy for accountability of the private health sector. As a physician, she has previously worked in HIV-prevention services among high-risk groups as a part of the AVAHAN programme in India since 2009, and continues to provide health services to the LGBTQIA+ community in Pune and Maharashtra through Project Accelerate.

K. Srinath Reddy is the president, Public Health Foundation of India (PHFI), and formerly headed the department of cardiology at the All India Institute of Medical Sciences, New Delhi. Under his leadership, PHFI has established five Indian Institutes of Public Health (IIPHs) to advance multidisciplinary public health education, research, health technologies and implementation support for strengthening health systems. He served as the first Bernard Lown Visiting Professor of Cardiovascular Health at the

Harvard School of Public Health (2009–13) and is presently an adjunct professor at Harvard University and Emory University. He has over 560 scientific publications. He is the first Indian to be elected to the National Academy of Medicine, USA. He was also president of the World Heart Federation (2013–15). He is a Padma Bhushan awardee.

Madhumitha Krishnan is a consultant Ayurveda paediatrician and CAPPA-certified childbirth educator (CCCE) based in Bengaluru. She works as consultant with CABHN, TDU, Bengaluru and runs a programme on introduction to Ayurveda dietetics and advanced Ayurveda dietetics. She works as a consultant paediatrician at multiple centres in Bengaluru and Hyderabad, handling cases of special children with an excellent track record of improving their quality of life. Madhumitha also works as an Ayurveda educator at KYM, Chennai.

Mekhala Krishnamurthy is senior fellow at the Centre for Policy Research (CPR) and associate professor of sociology and anthropology at Ashoka University. She is an ethnographer of the state and economy in contemporary India, and has researched and published extensively in the fields of health care and agriculture, especially on India's agricultural markets, their regional diversity, institutional complexity, regulatory life, and social and political dynamics. Her cross-sectoral interest centres on the people of the state and the everyday life of public institutions and systems. She leads the State Capacity Initiative at the CPR, which seeks to deepen and expand the understanding of the challenges and possibilities of building state capacity in democratic and federal India.

Pavitra Mohan is a community health physician, paediatrician and a public health practitioner. He is co-founder of Basic Health Care Services, a not-for-profit organization that provides low-cost, high-quality primary health-care services for the marginalized populations in south Rajasthan. Dr Mohan also serves as director of Health Services at Aajeevika Bureau, where he leads the designing and implementing of solutions for improving health of families that are dependent on labour and migration. Earlier, as senior health specialist at UNICEF India Country Office, he designed and led large-scale health programmes to improve maternal, newborn and child health in India. He earned his MBBS and MD in paediatrics from Delhi University and a master's in public health from the University of North Carolina at Chapel Hill. For his contribution to newborn health, he was inducted as a fellow of National Neonatology Forum of India in 2010. Recently, he has been awarded the prestigious Ashoka Fellowship for social entrepreneurship.

Purushottam M. Kulkarni is a demographer based in Bengaluru. He obtained a PhD degree in statistics from the Colorado State University and was a post-doctoral fellow in population studies at Brown University. He worked in various research and educational institutions in India and retired as professor of population studies at the Jawaharlal Nehru University. His areas of research interest are technical demography, fertility, reproductive and child health, sex ratio at birth, and population policies and programmes.

Rajib Dasgupta is professor and chairperson at the CSMCH, JNU. He was Fulbright Senior Research Fellow at Johns Hopkins Bloomberg School of Public Health (2010–11) and visiting professor at the University of Technology Sydney (2016). He is actively engaged with the national health policy initiatives and programme evaluations, and with the ongoing disease eradication/ elimination programmes. Widely published in national and international journals, he was managing editor of the *Indian Journal of Community Medicine* (2012–14) and is currently managing editor of the *Indian Journal of Public Health*. He is a regular commentator in international and national electronic and print media.

Ramani Atkuri is a graduate of the Christian Medical College, Vellore, where she also completed her MD in community medicine. Since then, she has been working with tribal and rural deprived communities in Odisha, Chhattisgarh and Madhya Pradesh. She also worked for ten years as a programme officer, health, UNICEF. Her interests include primary health care, especially maternal and childcare, issues of adult and child hunger, communicable diseases and health issues faced by migrants. She is also keenly interested in training. She believes that health care is much more than medical care, and that health is a deeply political issue.

Ritu Priya, professor at the Centre of Social Medicine and Community Health, Jawaharlal Nehru University, New Delhi, is a medical graduate and a community health researcher. The politics of knowledge between experts and laypeople, as well as between healing systems and traditions, are her exceptional contributions in public health. With a passion for democratizing, decolonizing and demystifying health and health care, she links epidemiology, popular culture, political economy and health systems analysis for contextually suited health systems development policy and planning. Urban health, nutrition and communicable diseases, Dalit and informal sector workers' health perceptions are specific themes studied using interdisciplinary and transdisciplinary research methodologies. Besides articles published in books and journals, she has an edited volume, *Dialogue on AIDS: Perspectives for the Indian Context*, and a book titled *Lok Swasthya Mein Samagrata Ki Khoj*. She has been adviser (public health planning) with the National Health Systems Resource Centre under the National Rural Health Mission, and member of advisory committees for the Planning Commission, Ministry of Health and Family Welfare, National AIDS Control Organization, Department/Ministry of AYUSH and the Indian Council for Medical Research. She is founder–member of the Trans-Disciplinary Research Cluster on Sustainability Studies and the founder–convenor of the Trans-Disciplinary Research Cluster on Plural Health Care at JNU.

Rohina Joshi heads the Global Health Program at the School of Population Health, University of New South Wales, and is senior recipient of the Australian National Heart Foundation Future Leader Fellowship and the UNSW Scientia Fellowship. Rohina's research and teaching aim to strengthen health systems, especially the health workforce and health information systems. She was awarded the Sax Institute Research Action Award for improving the quality of death certificates in the Philippines. She is a technical adviser for the Data for Health Initiative for the Mortality in India, established through verbal autopsy.

Shweta Marathe works as a health systems researcher at SATHI, Pune. After working with corporate hospitals for a couple of years, she switched to the NGO sector and has been with SATHI for the last eleven years. She coordinates SATHI's research division and leads/co-leads various research studies related to the functioning of the public health system, community nutrition and the private health-care sector. She is keen to conduct research to support advocacy and action towards policy change. Her research interest focuses on transformations in the private health-care sector in India. Please see https://www.researchgate.net/ for publications.

Sujatha Rao is a former union secretary of the Ministry of Health and Family Welfare, Government of India. An MA from Delhi University, Rao has an MPA from Harvard University, USA, was a Takemi fellow at the Harvard School of Public Health and the Gro Harlem Brundtland Senior Leadership fellow at HSPH. She was board member of The Global Fund, WHO and UNAIDS, the global advisory panel of the Bill and Melinda Gates Foundation; of the Public Health Foundation of India; was on the advisory board of the Ministerial Leadership Program of the Harvard School of

Public Health; of the Population Council, USA, AIIMS, Raipur, BSNL, etc. She is the author of *Do We Care?: India's Health System*, published by Oxford University Press in 2017.

Syeda Saiyidain Hameed is a feminist writer actively engaged in public affairs. She was a member of the National Commission for Women (NCW) from 1997 to 2000, and member of the Planning Commission of India from 2004 to 2014. In 1997, as member of the National Commission for Women, she toured the country and wrote extensively on atrocities and injustices faced by Indian women, with the objective of fulfilling the mandate of the NCW, namely, making systemic changes. In 2000 she wrote the first-ever report on Muslim women, *Voice of the Voiceless: Status of Muslim Women in India*. As member of the Planning Commission, she headed the areas of health, women and children, minorities, handloom and handicrafts, micro, medium and small enterprises, and the voluntary sector. She has a PhD in literature from the University of Alberta, Canada (1972), and was appointed lecturer first at the Lady Shri Ram College, New Delhi, and sessional lecturer at the University of Alberta, Canada. The next ten years saw her becoming the executive assistant to the minister of advanced education and manpower, Government of Alberta, Canada, and director of colleges and universities for the Alberta government. Returning to India in 1984, she devoted herself to writing and social activism, and served as a fellow at the Nehru Memorial Museum. She has engaged with several Indian and international civil society organizations in initiating pathbreaking changes. She is the founder of organizations such as Muslim Women's Forum, Women's Initiative for Peace in South Asia (WIPSA), South Asians for Human Rights (SAHR) and the Centre for Dialogue and Reconciliation. She is chair of the National Foundation of India and is on the governing board of, among others, The Hunger Project, ActionAid India and the Population Foundation of India.

T.S. Singh Deo is an Indian politician from Chhattisgarh. Currently, he is serving as a cabinet minister for health and family welfare, and medical education in the Chhattisgarh government. He has been actively engaged with evolving the policy approach and strategies for universal health care in the state. He was leader of Opposition in the fourth Vidhan Sabha of Chhattisgarh and served as chairman for the Chattisgarh State Finance Commission. Since 2008, he has been an elected member of the Chhattisgarh Legislative Assembly from Ambikapur, the capital of Surguja district, with which the Singh Deo dynasty has been associated for generations. He did his graduation in history from Hindu College, Delhi, and postgraduation from the Government Hamidia College, Bhopal.

T. Sundararaman was formerly executive director of the National Health Systems Resource Centre, New Delhi, and then served as professor and dean at the School of Health Systems Studies, Tata Institute of Social Sciences, Mumbai. A professor of internal medicine in JIPMER earlier, in 2002 he shifted to working full time with health systems strengthening. All along he has also been a health rights activists associated with people's health movements and recently completed a term as global coordinator of the People's Health Movement. His major public health contributions have been to the design and implementation of the National Rural Health Mission, and earlier of the Mitanin programme and health systems strengthening in Chhattisgarh.

Varnita Mathur is a software engineer with over twenty years of experience in the IT industry. She is passionate about data, its democratization and leveraging technology to improve data–driven decision-making. Her work focuses on biodiversity and health care, and exploring the interconnections between environment, animal and human health.

Vikram Patel is the Pershing Square Professor of Global Health at the Harvard Medical School. His work spans the areas of mental health problems, child development and adolescent health, in particular the use of community resources for assessment, prevention and recovery. He co-founded Sangath, an Indian NGO, which has won the MacArthur Foundation's International Prize for Creative and Effective Institutions and the WHO Public Health Champion of India award. He is a fellow of the UK Academy of Medical Sciences and was awarded an OBE. He was named as *Time* magazine's 100 most influential persons of the year in 2015 and was the 2019 laureate of the John Dirk Canada Gairdner Award in Global Health.

Vivekanand Jha is the executive director at the George Institute for Global Health, India, the chair of Global Kidney Health at Imperial College, London, and former president of the International Society of Nephrology. Prof. Jha is recognized as a global expert on kidney diseases. He currently leads research projects in more than ten countries. He is particularly interested in using multidisciplinary approaches and innovations to address the system level health and economic challenges posed to humanity by public-health threats through implementation research, particularly non-communicable diseases and environmental change.

About Samruddha Bharat Foundation

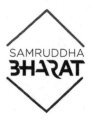

The Samruddha Bharat Foundation (SBF) strives to forge a resurgent and strong India that is a global superpower, a cosmopolitan beacon of democracy and accommodative of every Indian. It does so by constructively reshaping India's

▶ *Software* (transforming mass consciousness, public discourse, popular and social culture, education as well as by forging principled coalitions); and
▶ *Hardware* (reforming policies, institutions and governance to reorder India's polity, economy and society).

In breathing life into these goals, the SBF works closely with India's progressive parties, the nation's foremost thinkers, activists as well as a plethora of organizations and movements. The SBF thus serves as a clearing house for all progressive forces to collaborate in furthering the constitutional idea of India. For further details, see:

Website: www.samruddhabharat.in

Twitter: @SBFIndia

Facebook: Samruddha Bharat Foundation

Instagram: @SBFIndia